Paediatric Clinical Examination

Denis Gill MB, BSc, DCH, FRCP(I)
Professor of Paediatrics, Royal College of Surgeons in Ireland and
The Children's Hospital, Temple Street, Dublin

Niall O'Brien MB, DCH, FRCP(I)
Paediatrician with a special interest in Neonatology, National Maternity
Hospital, Holles Street and The Children's Hospital, Temple Street,
Dublin

CHURCHILL LIVINGSTONE
EDINBURGH LONDON MELBOURNE AND NEW YORK 1988

CHURCHILL LIVINGSTONE
Medical Division of Longman Group UK Limited

Distributed in the United States of America by
Churchill Livingstone Inc., 1560 Broadway, New
York, N. Y. 10036, and by associated companies,
branches and representatives throughout the world.

First published 1988
  Reprinted 1989
  Reprinted 1990

ISBN 0-443-03956-9

British Library Cataloguing in Publication Data
Gill, Denis
  Paediatric clinical examination.
  1. Children — Diseases — Diagnosis
  2. Physical diagnosis
  I. Title II. O'Brien, Niall
  618.92′00754   RJ50

Library of Congress Cataloging in Publication Data
Gill, Denis.
  Paediatric clinical examination.
  Bibliography: p.
  Includes index.
  1. Children — Medical examination. 2. Physical
diagnosis. I. O'Brien, Niall. II. Title.
[DNLM: 1. Physical Examination — in infancy &
childhood. WS 141 G475p]
RJ50.G55 1988   618.92′0075   87-34140

Produced by Longman Singapore Publishers (Pte) Ltd.
Printed in Singapore

To our children: Kieron, Daniel, Aisling, Meagan, Michael, Slaney, Eoin, Cliona, Helene and Aisling

Preface

This text was prepared on the basis of our perception of the need for a simple, unpretentious approach to clinical examination of children. Our objective was to produce a text which would be instructive, enjoyable and stimulating. The impetus arose from student criticism of teaching techniques of paediatric physical examination. We hope that our didactic approach will encourage students to examine children both thoroughly and thoughtfully.

We pay homage to our teachers and mentors, who may recognize some of their aphorisms, axioms and witticisms effortlessly regurgitated herein. We also thank our students for keeping us constantly on our toes and for catalysing us to produce this primer. We would welcome students' comments, criticisms and contributions.

Finally, we appreciate the support and patience of our respective wives, Margaret and Hélène. We must naturally acknowledge the experience and insight gained from observing our own children from cot to college.

Dublin, 1988

Denis Gill
Niall O'Brien

Acknowledgements

We could not have delivered the text without the tireless typing of Norma McEneaney, the photographic shots of Thomas Nolan, and the lively illustrations of Des Hickey; to all of them we are extremely grateful. We thank Professor Alan Browne for his view of the Hippocratic tradition.

Contents

1

Introduction

The text is aimed at undergraduate medical students taking their paediatric course and also at postgraduate doctors commencing their first post in paediatrics. Experience has taught us that paediatric residents frequently need to refresh and retrain themselves in child health and disease. The term 'student' refers therefore to both postgraduate and undergraduate students of paediatrics. Strange though it may seem, under and postgraduate education are interrelated. The medical graduate has an inherent obligation to remain a student for life. Our aims are to emphasize the important art of history taking both from parents and child, to guide in the elicitation and interpretation of physical signs in children of varying age, and to provide some sources of further information.

The doctor caring for little children needs to develop his observational and instinctual skills. Occasionally the combination of an observational clue plus an instinctual cue can result in 'instant diagnosis'. Throughout we wish to emphasize the value of attentive observation.

Our approach is essentially clinical, and will be confined largely to symptoms and signs. This does *not* purport to be a textbook of paediatrics and no effort is made to include descriptions of syndrome identification, clinical conditions, laboratory investigations, or treatment protocols. These can all be found in standard textbooks. Our objective is to expand

1

the first few chapters of the basic text into a child-centered clinical approach towards problem solving in paediatrics.

We believe that the simple but subtle skills of physical examination and history taking are essential if one is to be a dedicated doctor to children. Too many students spend inappropriate time in the library at the expense of being at the bedside. Our philosophy is that the student cannot examine too many babies, infants, or children. To know the abnormal, you must first know the normal.

We suspect that medical students may be exposed to a surfeit of unusual cases and conditions at the expense of more common and mundane problems. Remember that what is common is common, and that one must be versed in the usual to become good at the unusual.

We have elected to concentrate mainly on the newborn, infant and preschool child, for these are the ages of greatest change and most difficulty. The schoolchild is rational and reasonable, and can usually be examined as a 'mini-adult' in an organized fashion.

This text is written on the understanding that students taking paediatrics have had previous exposure to clinical methods. No effort is made, therefore, to define basic clinical terms such as, for example, crepitations, clubbing or chorea. Studded through the text are boxes containing special paediatric terminology with which the student may experience difficulty. Textbooks sometimes display disease in its most florid form. Insufficient emphasis may be placed on nuances of disease and degrees of disorder. Implicit in paediatrics is an ability to recognize subtle signs of sickness and to be able to say with some certainty that a baby is 'off' or an infant is 'ill'. Early recognition of problems facilitates early intervention and, hopefully, prevention of complications.

We trust that students will enjoy this primer and point out to us its deficits as well as their own problems. Paediatrics (doctoring of little people) should, above all, be pleasurable.

Think of your children's experience as being in a 'learning hospital' rather than a 'teaching hospital'.

Listen to and learn from children. And mimic their main attribute, that of a constantly questioning nature. Ask 'why?' over and over again.

- Look and you should see.
- Ask and you should be answered.

The basic requirements needed to acquire the clinical skills in paediatrics are the same as those for adult medicine in the Hippocratic tradition:

Clinical skill	Requirement
History taking	Education
Physical examination	Skill
Diagnosis	Inductive logic
Prognosis	Experience
Treatment	Knowledge

Sufficient incentive should be provided by the needs of children for good doctors, and by your need to pass your assessment. We do hope to transfer some of the skills required to examine children and to provide a flavour of the rewards to be obtained by good practice.

Recall at all times the ancient adage:

- I hear and forget
- I see and remember
- I do and understand.

'VETERINARY' PAEDIATRICS

By using the term 'veterinary' we are not attempting to be derogatory, but are trying to draw your attention to certain analogies between young children and animals. We also hope to persuade you to commence all examinations as veterinarians do — by listening and looking.

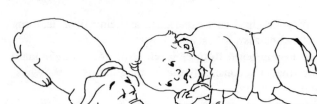

Fig. 1.1 'Veterinary Paediatrics': small children and animals share certain characteristics.

Some attributes shared by animals and small children are:
- they don't like being stared at
- they lie down when sick
- repeated food refusal is unusual
- they have limited ability to express themselves
- they adopt the position of comfort when well
- their survival instinct is strong.

Inspection and intuition are therefore important introductions to paediatric examination.

Some cynic has coined the term 'paediatric zoology' to describe the collection and study of rare cases and conditions within teaching hospitals!

AIMS AND OBJECTIVES IN PAEDIATRICS

Every department of child health will set its own course aims and objectives. In broad terms they will include the following main headings:

1. To teach the recognition and management of the well and ill infant and child.

2. To emphasize the importance of growth and development of both the normal and the sick child.

3. To provide a sound basic knowledge of child health and disease.

4. To enable the student to acquire sufficient skill to carry

out a full physical examination of a newborn infant, toddler, child and adolescent.

5. To demonstrate adequate medical, developmental, social and behavioural history taking from the parents or guardians of the child.

6. To stress the importance of the child's family and social background in relation to his well-being and illnesses.

7. To emphasize the importance of prevention in paediatrics; in particular this applies to immunization, nutrition and avoidance of accidents.

8. To demonstrate the relationship between genetic and environmental factors in the causation of malformation and of illness.

9. To provide an understanding of the handicapping conditions of childhood and of the services available for their amelioration.

The student should set himself the more straighforward and simple targets:

1. To be able to elicit and interpret findings from history and physical examination.

2. To be able to construct a reasonable differential diagnosis and problem list.

3. To be able to prepare plans for appropriate investigation and management.

4. To be able to communicate adequately with children and with their parents.

THE SEVEN AGES OF CHILDREN

Children change, grow, mature and develop. One's style and approach to physical examination will very much depend on the child's age, independence and understanding. The seven ages of children are:

- newborn, neonate: first month of life
- infancy: 1 month to 1 year

- toddler: 1 year to 3 years
- preschool child: 3–5 years
- schoolchild: 5–15 years
- child: 0–15 years
- adolescent: early 10–14 years
                              late 15–19 years.

Throughout the text the terms 'he', 'him', 'his', should be taken to be ambisextrous' and to refer to 'him' and 'her'. We reject the use of neuter 'it' in referring to children.

CHILDREN IN HOSPITAL

It has been said that the primary function of paediatricians is to discharge children from hospital. In developed countries the average inpatient stay has dropped steadily and now has a mean of 4–6 days. Indeed many children only stay 1–2 days. Students will need to be on their toes if they are to see and learn. About half of all admissions will be infants and toddlers — hence the importance where possible, of an omnipresent parent.

Parallel with reduced inpatient stay has been an increased use of day care, both for medical and surgical purposes. Many of the most interesting and complicated paediatric cases are to be found having various procedures in the plastic, orthopaedic, urological and neurosurgical units.

Why are children in hospital?
- for care of acute and chronic illnesses
- for surgery, acute and elective
- for investigative, therapeutic, and diagnostic procedures
- for multidisciplinary assessment, particularly if handicapped
- for their protection (in cases of serious nonaccidental injury)

- for observation (in behavioural and other disorders)
- for social reasons.

In the future much of paediatrics will be practiced on an 'ambulatory' basis — in the day ward, in the outpatient department and in the community clinic. During your paediatric course, visits to all these activities will be imperative. In addition, we recommend visits to child oriented general practices, institutes for the mentally and physically handicapped, and vaccination sessions.

Inner city children's hospitals tend to continue to have busy accident and emergency ('casualty') departments. In reality, a large proportion (as much as 50%) of the work of these departments relates to primary care problems, that is, medical conditions that should be handled in the community. We urge students to avail of the opportunity to see the common problems in practice — respiratory infections, infectious illnesses, minor injuries, rashes, vague symptoms, etc, in the Accident and Emergency department. Remember that while leukaemia, nephrotic syndrome, and epiglottitis may be relatively common conditions in hospital practice, they are distinctly rare in general practice. The general practitioner is more likely to encounter iron deficiency anaemia, urinary tract infection and viral 'croup' than any of the above.

By their nature, children's hospitals tend to have a disproportionate collection of curiosities and congenital disorders. Remember our rules:

- first know the normal
- then know variants of normal
- then know abnormality, noting that:
- normality and abnormality are close allied, and thin partitions do their bounds divide.

Some 5–7% of children are admitted to hospital annually, and some 50% of children have been in hospital by the age of 7 years. Observe the effects of hospitalization on children. Note the trauma of separation if a parent cannot be present.

Learn of the efforts that are now being made to mitigate the effects of hospitalization on vulnerable children through preparation, play, parental accommodation, painting and above all pleasant hospital people from porters to professors. While nurses are nearly always nice and doctors do their best, students should be simple, straight and considerate in their approach to children. Remember the words of Marcus (aged 6) who wrote 'even nasty people are nice when you're ill'.

THREE PILLARS OF DIAGNOSIS

Medical diagnosis rests on the traditional tripod of history, physical examination and investigation. Paediatric problem solving rests heavily on history, partly on examination (observation) and partly on investigation. A carefully taken and properly recorded history is the clinical keystone. The history should give prime emphasis to the mother's worries and reasons for bringing the child to the doctor. Physical examination, with its techniques, tricks and tribulations is

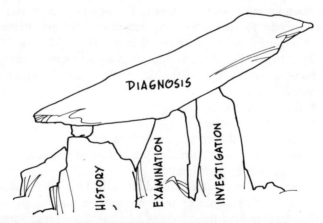

Fig. 1.2 The three pillars of diagnosis are history, physical examination and investigation.

described in detail in other parts of this text. The results of examination need to be recorded in a standard legible style with due emphasis of relevant negative findings. The brief designation O/E NAD (on examination, nothing abnormal detected), is inadequate for undergraduate purposes.

With experience, a thorough examination of infants and children can be completed in a short time. Parents are very reassured by doctors who do a thorough examination, not merely confining themselves to the presenting part, be that a sore ear or a limp. There is simply no substitute for examining lots of normal children. Know the normal and deviations ·can be subsequently recognized. Today's parents (of smaller families) want to know that their children are normal and if not, what is the matter.

- History is the keystone.
- Examine the whole child.
- see lots of children.

We shall not refer to investigation in this book, but rather refer you to your standard text.

> 'I seek a method by which the teachers teach less and learners learn more.'
>
> Comenius (1630)

2

History taking

> 'A smart mother makes often a better diagnosis than a poor doctor'
>
> August Bier (1861–1949)

LISTENING TO MOTHERS

The most important attribute of any good doctor is to be a good listener. Listen carefully to mothers and note what they say. History is the vital cornerstone of paediatric problem

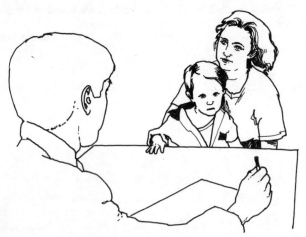

Fig. 2.1 Listen attentively to mother.

solving. More important information is often gathered from a good history than from physical examination and laboratory investigation.

The first important ground rule in history taking is: *mother is right until proved otherwise.* Mothers are, by and large, excellent observers of their offspring and make good interpreters of their problems when sick. Even the most ill-educated mother will often surprise you by her intuition. She may not know what's wrong but she certainly knows something is wrong. If a mother says 'I think my baby can't hear properly', the onus is on the doctor to corroborate or negate that statement.

In our view no one can replace the mother in providing an accurate and thorough description of the child and his complaints. Fathers will vary in their expertise, but often lack the information, insight and instinct that a good mother can provide. While the principle that mother is usually right prevails, the corollary must be that fathers can be off cue and off course. However, the modern day domesticated father is improving. Other caretakers — guardians, aunts, house-mothers — will vary widely in their knowledge of the child. We have been impressed by the inhibitory nature of some grandparents' presence at initial interviews and history taking.

At the outset it is important to try to establish a good rapport with the mother. Allow her to understand that you are more concerned with what she has to say than what Dr. X has suggested. Make sure you understand her idiom and her concerns. A useful opening question is: 'what do you yourself think really is the cause of his trouble?' or 'do you have any views as to what is wrong with him?'

These questions may lead you in the right direction. Alternatively, they may be important to negate following examination and investigation. Get into the habit of quoting verbatim from mother. Mothers frequently make statements whose importance, if not noted and recorded during history taking, may be subsequently lost. We have both the experience of saying to ourselves: 'if only I had listened to that mother; she was trying to tell me what was wrong'.

Students can unquestioningly accept a mother's complaints about her child without asking her to define her terms. Terms such as diarrhoea or vomiting require definition. Does diarrhoea mean frequent stools, semi-formed stools, offensive stools? Do you (or mother) know the normal frequency of stool passage? Is it reasonable to expect a single teenage parent to know children? What does the term 'hyperactivity' mean to you — are not all children active to varying degrees?

Listen to mother talking:
- what are her worries?
- what does she think?
- quote verbatim
- understand her idiom
- ask her to define her terms (what do you mean by . . . . . ?).

You need to establish that you are both talking about the same thing, be it croup, anorexia or breath-holding. You need also to learn her local idiom or slang (the penis may be referred to as the private parts, willy or johnny for example). In our hospital the residents have come to learn that when mothers say that the baby is 'lobbing and lying', they mean something serious is wrong. Australian mothers may state that the infant is 'crook'.

One needs to know the questions which produce the desired answers. A good opening ploy is 'tell me about your baby' and then simply let the mother talk. As you gain experience you will learn the important pointers and know when to interject succinct questions without interrupting her flow.

The student must of course take thorough notes interspersed with pithy quotations or spicy titbits. In time you'll learn how to cut corners, how to proceed down diagnostic avenues, or how to recognize important cues. Learn through history taking (receiving) to be a good listener — to parents primarily, but also to your better teachers as they elicit clinical histories.

Always ask the parents to relate the sequence of events leading to the present complaints. A suitable start might be: 'When was he last well? Which came first, the cough or the wheeze? In what way has he changed?' In eliciting the history of a convulsion, details of the time, place, surroundings, stimuli, etc. are of vital importance.

You will need also to obtain a general knowledge of the child. What sort of fellow is he? Is he active? Has he much energy? Is he outgoing, sociable? How does he sleep? Is school progress satisfactory? Is he developing normally? Whose side of the family does he resemble?

Let mothers talk:
- tell me about your baby
- what sort of fellow is he?
- when was he last well?
- tell me what happened.

Patients also appreciate a doctor who gives them individual attention and whose time is devoted to them (even though he may be in a hurry). Listen and you will hear. Time spent on history taking will be well repaid. Try to ensure that your written notes reflect adequately the time taken and interest shown. Some mothers do 'beat about the bush' dragging in all sorts of irrelevancies. With experience you will learn how to conduct and interrupt such garrulous gabblers.

Any of your standard texts and tutors will cite examples of how to fully explore a symptom, such as cough or pain.

When does it occur?
How long has he had it?
Can you describe it?
What brings it on?

Does anything relieve it?
How long does it last?
What is its pattern and periodicity?
Are there any associated symptoms?
What does he do when he has it?
What have you done about it?

This will necessarily be followed by a careful and thorough exploration of the relevant system, and then by a systems review. With time and experience, systems reviews tend to abbreviate and to become more precise. There is nothing special or different in paediatrics about the necessity of obtaining an adequate past history, family history, and social history. Awareness of the child's place in the family, relationship with parents, siblings and peers is crucial in obtaining a broad view of the child. So many of today's illnesses have social and behavioural overtones that the importance of the holistic view cannot be overemphasized.

A knowledge of the family's socioeconomic status, present financial situation, housing, and employment is vital. Are the parents married, separated, cohabiting? Is the mother single? In some cases of handicap or metabolic disorder it will be prudent to enquire cautiously about consanguinity.

CUE WORDS

Computers accept key words; students ought to look out for *cue words* when taking histories. By cue words we mean simple statements, hidden in histories, which may be diagnostically alerting. Let us cite a few examples.

1. Cue: 'She does not like bread or biscuits.'
    Think: Could this be gluten enteropathy?
2. Cue: 'He just loves salt; he even licks it from things.'
    Question: Has he a salt losing state?

3. Cue: 'He's hungry after he vomits.'
   Answer: This is suggestive of mechanical vomiting, whether due to pyloric stenosis or gastro-oesophageal reflux.
4. Cue: 'He's always drinking, he'll drink anything, he'll even drink from toilet bowls.'
   Response: This sounds like true polydipsia.
5. Cue: 'I don't know where all the food goes.'
   Comment: When referred to a relatively inactive infant this statement may suggest a malabsorptive state, for example cystic fibrosis.

Mothers may, of course, unintentionally deceive. A common complaint is: 'I can't get him to eat anything'. And there in front of you sits a solemn, pudgy infant sucking on a bottle containing a melange of milk, rusks, and maybe tea. In a similar vein, the seemingly contradictory statements, 'but he eats nothing doctor' followed rapidly by 'he never stops going' are frequently encountered. They usually reflect the overactive (and perhaps underdisciplined) toddler who is 'addicted to the bottle' and is consuming excessive carbohydrate by day and night.

A SAMPLE HISTORY

To obtain the right answers any detective must know how to ask (and frame) the right questions. This simple maxim applies to any system; nowhere is it more pertinent than in taking a history of a fit or convulsion. In any convulsion one needs to know as much as possible, about the child, his environment and the surrounding circumstances.

However, by way of example of a thorough history we have chosen the questioning of a mother whose child is wetting the bed (enuretic). This common complaint, source of much maternal irksomeness but often a dearth of medical interest, exemplifies the value of detailed and diligent history taking.

What age is he?

Where does he come in the family?

When did the bed wetting commence?

How frequently does he wet?

Does he wet by day?

How long can he retain his urine by day?

Does he have a good stream?

Has he had any kidney infections?

When was he dry by day?

Was dryness achieved easily or with difficulty?

Has he his own bed?

Does he wake when he wets?

Does he waken more than once per night?

Is he in nappies at night?

Who changes the sheets?

Have you inside toilets?

What have you done about wetting?

Does he want to be dry?

Has he had any dry nights?

What was his best dry period?

Is he dry when away?

Have you lifted him?

Have you restricted his fluids?

Have you reprimanded or punished him?

How does he get on at home and in school?

Have medication or alarms been tried?

Did any of his siblings wet at night?

Were either of you (his parents) wet when children?

How does the wetting affect him?

How does the wetting bother you?

This may seem a ream of questions but with experience they can trip off the tongue promptly and build up a picture of the child and his problem. Bed wetting is one of those complaints where it can be useful to see the child and mother both together and separately.

Similar interrogation in depth can be constructed for a whole variety of symptoms from fits to fainting to feeding difficulties. There is simply no substitution for a thorough history, properly phrased and fully recorded, in diagnosing childhood disorders. Try writing one for asthma, abdominal pain or anaemia. Think of a suitable programme of questions one might feed into a computer and have the parents perform themselves while awaiting consultation.

Feeding history

Feeding is such an intrinsic part of infancy, and feeding problems so common that a good history on feeding pattern and content is crucial. Too many doctors when presented with a feeding problem change the milk. The problem does not usually lie in the milk but in management of feeding and in the mother-infant relationship (harmonious or otherwise?). A detailed feeding history is vital if one is going to be able to discuss diet with today's allergy conscious mothers.

Was the baby bottle or breast fed? If *breast fed*, what was the duration of exclusive breast feeding? Was this a satisfying experience for mother and baby? How often did she feed? Was he content? Were there any problems? How did he sleep, feed and gain? Did she feed on demand or to some sort of schedule? Was she complementing the breast milk with anything else?

If *bottle fed*, was he fed on formula or unmodified cow's milk? Which formula did he receive? How was it prepared? What volume did he take each feed and how long did he take over it? Frequency of feeds? Total daily intake? Any additives (iron or vitamins) given with milk? Duration of exclusive milk feeding?

Weaning

At what age were solids first introduced? Which solids? How were they administered — by spoon or in bottle? At what age were gluten-containing foods first given? Had he any preferences? When could he manage lumpy food?

Allergies

Any known food allergies? Why do you think he is allergic to that substance? Does he suck well? Does he swallow well? What stops him feeding? Is it, for example, satiety, sleepiness or breathlessness? Were there weaning problems? How did you two get on? Did your husband assist with bottle feeding? Do you feed him every time he cries? Do you give him drinks of water?

If all these questions fail to sort out the problem, one may have to resort to the request — show me how you do it please.

Students can with benefit spend time doing nursing duties — changing, washing, holding and above all feeding babies. Learn by doing.

In conclusion, good history taking is the hallmark of the good student of paediatrics.

A *full paediatric history* will enquire along the following general lines:

pregnancy
delivery
perinatal events
feeding practice
developmental progress
immunizations
infectious diseases
accidents and injuries
hospital admissions and operations
allergies

minor illnesses
medications
serial heights and weight, if known
school progress
travel.

During the taking of the history, preferably in relaxed surroundings, the opportunity should arise to observe how the child separates from the parent, how creatively and independently he plays, and occasionally how expressively he draws.

The whole history and nothing but the whole history:
- the full facts
- the precise sequence of complaints
- changes noted since onset of illness.

LET THE CHILDREN SPEAK

While we repeatedly emphasize the value and importance of maternal history of her child's complaints, don't forget the

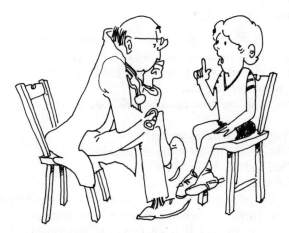

Fig. 2.2 Let the children speak!

child. He may be very anxious to tell you his story and may have a useful contribution to make. Oftentimes, especially if he's verbally precocious and outgoing, or if he has a chronic condition and much experience of hospital, he may express himself remarkably lucidly. Children need to be heard and be seen to be noticed. He has a viewpoint which he is frequently eager to express. Children over 5 years should be asked to give their account of events with parental corroboration of certain points.

If he's reticent, shy or mute don't push him. He may talk later. Allowing him to draw himself, his family, their home may be revealing to those with psychological insight. Use of a tape recorder, or even a video (if your department of Child Health is well equipped) can be useful particularly in exploring behavioural or conduct problems.

Make sure you know the child's pet name as well as his given name. Laurence may be called 'Larry', Robert 'Bobby' and Catherine 'Katie'. In addition, the child recorded as Patrick Joseph, may in fact be called 'Junior'.

TALKING TO PARENTS

While it is not our remit to discuss communication with parents, a few words on this topic seem pertinent. Good listening is contributory to learning, good communication is the key to cooperative caring.

Parents of ill children broadly seek four degrees of information:

1. What is it? What is wrong?
2. What caused it? How did it happen?
3. What will be the outcome?
4. Will it happen again?.

Clearly the answers to the above questions will considerably depend on whether the child's disorder is an acute one (e.g. meningitis) or whether it is an inherited abnormality (e.g.

cleft palate). It is evident that one has difficulty responding to questions 2, 3 and 4 if one cannot answer question 1. Students should be reticent about discussing causes and consequences with parents until they possess the appropriate acumen and authority. Finally, don't forget the unvoiced (fifth) question — is it leukaemia, or cancer, or some lethal familial trait?

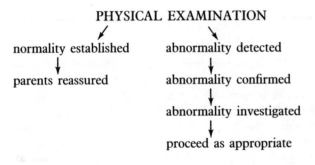

PHYSICAL EXAMINATION

normality established

↓

parents reassured

abnormality detected

↓

abnormality confirmed

↓

abnormality investigated

↓

proceed as appropriate

3

Approaching children

THE APPROACH CODE

The first rules in approaching any child are very similar to those for crossing the road — stop, listen, look, then use your senses. The first approach is a hands off one — *stop*. Allow the child to look at you and, in so far as he can, decide you are a person to be trusted. Let him look at you as you talk to his mother. Take your time, make no sudden moves (for you may frighten a fretful toddler) and be in no hurry to

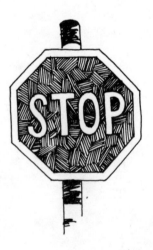

Fig. 3.1 Stop!

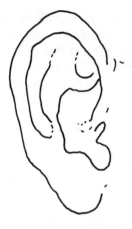

Fig. 3.2 Listen!

examine the child. Even better, let him play in your presence. Approach cautiously, be nice, utter reassuring sounds.

Listen to the mother. Children may come to the clinic, surgery or hospital in the company of a variety of caretakers, (mother, father, guardian, foster-parent, nurse, relative). In our view, there is no substitute for the mother. She knows her child. The guiding principle in listening is: mother is usually right until or unless proved otherwise. We have expanded on this in the section on history taking. At the same time you may have the opportunity to listen to the child talk, relate to his mother, and to note his breathing, cough, stridor (if present) and other auditory phenomena such as his cry.

Then *look*. Look at both mother and child. Is he sick or

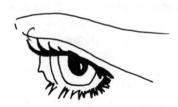

Fig. 3.3 Look!

well? Is he normal or abnormal? Does he resemble his parents? Always look at children without staring or looking too closely at them. Some toddlers share attributes with certain animals who do not like being stared at. Any instinctual clues? One must teach students to observe. Any observational cues?

'Learn to see things.'

Leonardo da Vinci

The approach code:
- stop
- listen
- look
- use your other senses.

Children are best approached in *their* position of comfort — lying flat in infancy, sitting on their mother's knee in toddlerhood, on their own two feet when of school age. Leave undressing to later — removal of clothes can be a threatening manoeuvre. Explain what you are about to do and be reassuring repeatedly. Don't lie the child down until you have to — he's very vulnerable in this position. Keep his mother close at hand. Always leave unpleasant procedures — throat examination, rectal examination — until the very last and don't do unless you feel they will be contributory.

Learn by listening to mothers, examining their children and then reading the chart. Too often students first read the notes and then go in search of what they are supposed to find. Students should at times take the opportunity of divesting their white coats — white coats bring needles and tests.

Never examine the presenting part only. From your earliest days train yourself to be thorough, and to be a generalist as opposed to a systems specialist. Remember one of the basic axioms — the good doctor treats the whole person, not just the sore belly or foot.

In summary, the best approach to infants and toddlers is

to begin examination with a *strict no touch technique*. Be a good looker.

In small infants *inspection* (of colour, breathing, activity, etc.) can be the key to diagnosis. Physical signs are frequently less florid in sick infants than they are in sick adults; students tend to be well trained in the arts of palpation and percussion, at the expense of inspection. We would agree with the words of Sir Dominic Corrigan (1853): 'the trouble with many doctors is not that they do not know enough but that they do not see enough'. Remember the importance of nonverbal communication. When you have looked, describe what you see. It is strange how difficult it can be to translate the observations into words. To say for example 'funny looking kid' (a pejorative term objectionable to some) without being able to describe what is 'funny' is ludicrous. The road to diagnosis in many dermatological problems is to set down in words (of English or literate Latin) what one sees. All too often the descriptive terms elude the student and he jumps at diagnoses like a salmon at flies.

Syndrome spotting is in the eye and mental computer of the beholder. Students need not be syndrome spotters. However, they should be able to recognize Down's syndrome, obvious congenital abnormalities, or significant dysmorphism.

First know the normal. Then the abnormal or different may become apparent. Ask yourself — what's odd about this face? Then describe in simple terms those relevant features — wide eyes, low set ears, upturned nose, arched palate, which contribute to your suspicions.

You should try to examine as much with your eyes as with your hands. You should also try to listen to the child 'speaking with his body' — noting that many childhood physical complaints have a background behavioural basis.

Use your other senses — touch, smell, taste (occasionally) to aid in diagnosis. These we will expand upon later. The child's doctor needs to be gentle of touch (cold hands — warm heart theorizing just will not do), to be able to extemporize (in other words do what you can when you can and not to adhere to a rigid, regimented approach to examination), but to be thoroughly sensitive and sensible.

It will be frequently necessary to humour the baby or to distract an infant's attention when attempting examination. The distraction tricks (commonsense really!) described below may help.

Play with babies, infants and children
Tickle babies (tickles appear at 3 months)
Play 'peek-a-boo'
Blow 'raspberries' at babies
Blow on their faces (they quite like this)
Allow toddlers to play with the examining instruments.
Give infants something to hold
Get mother to dangle an attractive toy or bright light
Talk nonsense/rubbish to young children — they've quite a good sense of humour and may think you're a likeable idiot.

> 'You can do anything with children if you only play with them'
>
> Otto von Bismarck
> (19th century)

Shake hands with children; curiously even toddlers may appreciate this formality. Hopefully you have allowed him to establish eye contact with you; social sensory contact may facilitate you in applying your examining hands. In other words, before you start, try to strike a rapport.

Before proceeding to discuss detailed physical examination of different ages and various parts of children, we would remind you of the four Cs of clinical examination which you should aim to achieve:

- confidence   — of child in you
                    (and you in yourself)
- competence   — in handling children

- completeness — of examination
- collation   — can you sum up and draw
                  conclusions from what you've
                  found?

THINGS NOT TO DO

Do not get the *sex* of the child wrong. This is understandably upsetting to parents. They begin to wonder if is it their child you are talking about. Never refer to a child as '*it*'. This is a frequent failing, sure to raise the ire of certain colleagues and examiners.

Never handle a child *roughly*. Gentleness must be the hall-mark of a good child's doctor. Apley used to preach:. 'It's my fault if the child cries'. One need not go so far as this, but must attempt not to cause distress during physical examination.

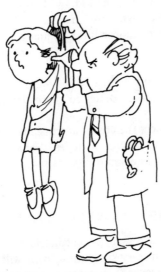

Fig. 3.4 Don't handle children roughly.

Do not speak derogatively in front of children. Even little ears are more attuned to doctor's talk than you may think.

Never refer to a child as a 'FLK' (funny looking kid) in front of the parents or without first seeing the parents. The term 'dysmorphic' might be more appropriate.

Do not drop the baby, they can be slippery, wriggly creatures, especially if covered in vernix caseosa. Our recent experience of a student dropping a baby (fortunately without harm) when demonstrating the Moro reflex to examiners was salutary.

Do not use *potentially worrying terms* in front of parents without explaining them. The term 'pyloric tumour' may seem innocuous to you. However, to the layman, tumour implies cancer. Similarly, we have given the diagnosis 'benign recurrent haematuria' to parents with explanation and reassurance, without realizing that some of them had interpreted the word 'benign' to imply that the urinary blood was coming from a benign cancer of the kidney. It is often prudent to tell parents of children who are anaemic — 'of course, it's not leukaemia'. Fear of cancer lurks in many a parental mind, at times and occasions when it never occurs to their attending doctors.

Do not misjudge the child's *age* — children are remarkably sensitive on this score. Better to overestimate than to underestimate age.

Do not disrespect the child's intrinsic *modesty* — which will vary between and within societies. Some children will not mind being fully undressed; others may need explanation or a compromise.

POINT TO THE PART WHICH PAINS

Pain is a common reason for paediatric consultation. Clearly the bulk of the history concerning pain will be sought from the parents. However, you must always ask the child to try to describe *his* pain.

The preschool child will certainly lack the vocabulary and communication skills to describe his pains, but can surely point them out. So ask him to show you the spot which pains. He can often pinpoint the appropriate place.

The older child should be asked to describe his pain, always checking with the parent his accuracy and veracity. A good mother will frequently coax the child without being asked: 'it's your pain, try to tell the doctor about it'.

Where is the pain?

Show me where it is?

What is it like?

What do you do when you get it?

Does it make you cry?

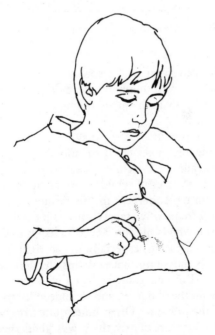

Fig. 3.5 Ask the child to point to the part which pains.

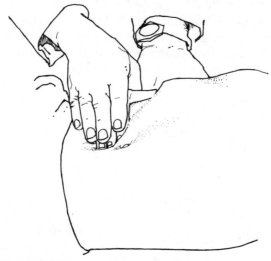

Fig. 3.6 Small children may allow you to palpate the abdomen over their own hand.

If the child can point to the spot, this should be reflected in your notes — 'left temporal headache' rather than just 'headache', or 'pain both upper thighs at night' rather than merely 'limb pains'.

A toddler or preschool child may resist abdominal examination. In the first instance distraction techniques may be tried. If these fail, use the child's hand to guide yours around the abdomen. A fretful child may allow you to assess abdominal pain or tenderness in this fashion.

One not infrequently meets the child with recurrent abdominal pain who is 'jumpy' and who seems to demonstrate tenderness on palpation, especially in the right iliac fossa. If in doubt as to the significance of this 'tenderness' a useful ploy is to say, 'I'm first going to listen with my stethoscope'. Lay it gently on the abdomen and do indeed listen but gradually increase the pressure. Often times quite firm pressure can be tolerated where previously there was 'tenderness'.

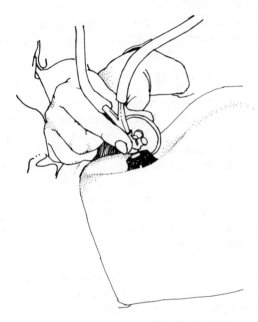

Fig. 3.7 Using the stethoscope to assess abdominal tenderness.

The child whose pain moves about in erratic fashion crossing anatomical boundaries and disobeying dermatomes needs to be taken with a grain of salt. By converse the child whose pain wakes him from his sleep, disturbs pleasurable activities or causes him to cry, needs to be heeded.

Unwillingness to move or use a limb may suggest pain therein. Dislike of being handled is typical of meningism. Pleuritic pain may be evident only splinting of one side of the chest — which is an infrequent, subtle sign missed even by experienced paediatricians. Small children have similarities with pets — when sick or sore they lie down without having to be told to do so.

'The only time children tell the truth is when they are in pain'
Bill Cosby

We don't agree entirely with the above statement, but do accept the sentiment that childhood pain is not figmentary.

PUTTING IT TOGETHER

Insofar as undergraduate students are concerned, diagnosis per se is not important. What is important is the ability to take a thorough history, elicit the relevant physical signs following examination, and attempt to interpret them. On the basis of the history and physical findings, the student may be able to construct a diagnosis, or a series of possible diagnoses.

Students must be prepared to write down their findings for public scrutiny. One can afford to be wrong as a student and learn from these mistakes. Being wrong may be a dent to one's doctoring dignity once qualified — doctors like to surround themselves with an aura of omniscience. In our opinion we should be more often prepared to say 'I don't know, but I'll look it up'. Students could usefully cultivate the practice of writing down things they don't understand, or findings whose explanation is unclear (what, for example is the physiology of yawning?), and of seeking the answers.

One should attempt to come to conclusions on the completion of history and physical examination. For example:

Problems: 1. Febrile convulsion
2. Follicular tonsillitis
3. Innocent murmur

It may be useful to add a postscript —

Mother's worries: 1. Brain damage
2. Nephew died of meningitis

and to deal with these prior to discharge.

If less sure of one's conclusions the 'bottom line' may read:

Impression: 1. Failure to thrive
2. Possible anaemia
3. Consider malabsorption

Note: Small, poor parents; no previous measurements.

It should be stated that differential diagnosis tends to play a less important part in paediatrics than in adult medicine, in that many childhood illnesses are straightforward uncomplicated entities compared to the complicated, cumulative, degenerative conditions of adulthood. Nonetheless one may have to consider and construct a differential diagnosis for diffuse lymphadenopathy, polyarthritis, acute encephalopathy, ataxia, haematuria, and many other clinical conditions.

Today's computer literate students may like the *key word approach*, writing down the important positive findings plus relevant negative findings and attempting to compute an answer:

erythematous rash
Raynaud's phenomenon
pauciarticular arthritis
alopecia
weight loss
swollen parotid gland.

The above example suggests a connective tissue disorder.

In recording the physical findings of children with multiple or chronic disorders, the problem based approach has much to recommend it. Below is an example from the notes of a child with spina bifida.

Problem	*Plan*
myelomeningocele	repaired after birth
hydrocephalus, ventriculo-peritoneal shunt	check function
moderate scoliosis	physiotherapy, posture
constipation	discuss diet, nursing
urinary incontinence	self catheterization?
short stature	no action
lower limb paralysis	physiotherapy, walking devices

The list could be extended further, but we hope you have got the message. Detection and diagnosis of problems is only useful if it can lead to a plan of action for their improvement.

I DON'T KNOW

Teach thy tongue to say:

> 'I do not know'

> Maimonides (1135–1204)

Doctors like to surround themselves with an aura of omniscience (how many doctors will consult a text in front of patients?). Students are not expected to know everything. If asked a question of which you don't know the answer, be prepared to say so rather than hazarding guesses. But you must later be prepared to look for the answer, solution or information. Or to ask the appropriate people to help you in finding out. A constantly questioning mind will serve you well during your career. The back pages of this text could well be filled with questions seeking answers. Above all don't be shy in asking. Simple questions often provide fascinating answers.

4

Examination at different ages

'Paediatrics is a specialty bound by age and not by system'.

NEWBORN

The great majority of newborn infants have had a normal intrauterine existence, a normal delivery, are in good condition at birth and are physically normal. However, there is a considerable variation in size and shape and appearance within the normal, which depends on parental, familial, genetic and ethnic factors. The foundation stone of paediatric medicine is only laid when the student has personally examined a large number of normal neonates, infants, toddlers, preschool and older children. The message therefore, is know the normal spectrum.

Delivery room

All newborns should be examined at birth to observe the general condition and to rule out major anomalies. The Apgar score is valuable because it determines whether resuscitation is necessary or not, and is internationally accepted. A poor score (< 5) at 5 minutes appears to relate to long term development. Examination of the cord for a single artery is of some value as a clue to the possibility of as yet hidden abnormalities. Having established that the infant does not require special or intensive care, and is overtly normal, the parents are accordingly informed.

Apgar score

Sign	Score		
	0	1	2
Colour	Blue, pale	Pink trunk Blue extremities	Pink all over
Heart rate	Absent	< 100	> 100
Reflex irritability	None	Grimace	Cry
Tone, activity	Limp	Some limb flexion	Active movement
Respiratory effort	Absent	Slow, irregular	Good strong cry

Postnatal ward

A further examination is usually carried out on the third day at which time the infant is almost unrecognizable from the one examined at delivery — skin nice and pink, head assuming normal shape, hair combed, and feeding well. The examination at this stage is much more detailed. The mother, and, if possible, the father should be present. Explanation should be offered as the examination proceeds and each test described as it is being performed. The mother is particularly influenced by the appearance of her baby — to include size (is he in normal centiles), facial appearance, colour and texture of skin, bruising, abrasions, scratch marks, rashes and subconjunctival haemorrhage. The latter condition is easily understood if the mother has suffered the same as a result of labour.

Blotchy erythematous rash is common; this is almost certainly erythema toxicum. Peeling of the skin that has been exposed to meconium is normal. This can be confirmed by discolouration of the cord stump and the presence of stained finger nails. Finger nails are often long and though soft can cause scratch marks. The toenails often appear to be ingrowing and this is of no consequence.

Jaundice is best observed in the sclera, skin and mucous

membranes, preferably in good daylight. Always switch off phototherapy unit lights when attempting to determine jaundice. We believe that it remains good practice (though fallible), to attempt to determine the degree of jaundice clinically. But always measure serum bilirubin of jaundiced infants. Phototherapy can induce the 'bronzed baby' syndrome.

Head and face

As the appearance of the baby is of concern to the mother, inspection and examination of the head and face should be carried out first. Local trauma is common and includes caput succadeneum and moulding, minor abrasions of the scalp, forceps marks, nonspecific facial bruises, subconjunctival haemorrhage and occasionally cephalhaematoma. In general, these conditions resolve spontaneously within the first week with the notable exception of cephalhaematoma which will calcify and resolve within 2–3 months. Cephalhaematoma is most commonly found over the parietal bone and confined to the edges. Occasionally both parietal bones are involved. Rarely the condition can involve the occipital bone when the possibility of an encephalocele should be considered.

Asymmetry of the face may occasionally be due to a transient seventh cranial nerve paresis which nearly always results from a forceps delivery. Head shape varies considerably during the first week. Marked moulding with caput occurs in some. Intrauterine pressure (when infant is in breech position) may produce an elongated head with protruberance of the occiput. Deflection, giving rise to face presentation, may be associated with severe bruising and oedema of the face, eyelids and lips. Chvostek's sign (tapping the facial nerve → twitching of the perioral muscle) is a normal finding in the newborn.

Plagiocephaly is not an uncommon finding related to intrauterine position. The head is skewed slightly or noticeably.

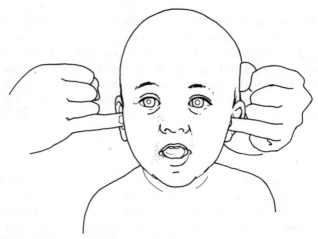

Fig. 4.1 Demonstrating plagiocephaly.

The simple trick of placing one finger on each ear of the forward looking head will demonstrate plagiocephaly readily.

The anterior fontanelle is normally open and can vary from 1 cm to 4 or 5 cm in diameter. Cranial sutures are usually mobile and the posterior fontanelle may accept a finger tip.

Ears

Can be of different shape and size and the amount of cartilage can vary. A low set ear where the top of the pinna is below a horizontal line from the outer canthus does *not* make a syndrome. Neither does the presence of preauricular ear tags.

Mouth

The shape of the mouth varies and a slanting lower jaw only reflects intrauterine head posture. Look for presence of a tooth, examine gums anteriorly and posteriorly to exclude ranula or cyst, check the size and shape of tongue.

The frenum linguae extends from the under-surface of the tongue to the floor of the mouth and is present in all children. Surgery on the frenum may rarely be required if there is interference with tongue protrusion or with growth of tongue tip. The soft palate and uvula should be observed.

Come to terms: head

frontal bossing:	= prominence of forehead, i.e. part of frontal bone
craniotabes:	= soft compressible skull bones

Come to terms: skull shapes

scaphocephaly	= boat shaped head (long, narrow)
macrocephaly	= large head (synonym = megalencephaly)
microcephaly	= very small head
plagiocephaly	= parallelogram (skew) head
turricephaly	= tall head (synonym = acrocephaly)
brachycephaly	= flat head (short head)
synostosis	= (premature fusion of adjacent bones)
trigonocephaly	= triangular shaped head

Eyes

Oedema of the eyelids is common, more particularly in the preterm. Bruising may also be present. Because of the oedema, opening the eyes may be difficult; if the examiner holds the infant in the upright or prone position, in most cases the eyes open. Look for conjunctival haemorrhage, clear cornea, evidence of cataract. Compare eye size and if in doubt palpate the eyes for size and eyeball pressure. Squint is common, though rarely paralytic in which case the 6th cranial nerve is usually involved. Accumulation of lacrimal fluid with secondary infection is extremely common and results usually from incomplete drainage of the nasolacrimal duct. If there is a lot of pus present, a specific infection such as gonococcal opthalmia should be considered.

Respiratory system

The respiratory system is best examined by observation. Observation of the colour of the infant's lips, mucosa and skin, and observation of respiratory rate and effort is infinitely more important than percussion and auscultation. Observation should include the rate of respiration (normally 30–50 per minute at rest), the rhythm of respiration and the work of respiration. Normal newborn respiration is quiet, effortless and predominantly diaphragmatic. There is more abdominal than chest movement.

Respiratory problems are common in the newborn and will be manifest by tachypnoea, increased respiratory effort and cyanosis. The infant may develop retraction, recession and variable respiratory rhythm. The students should comment on chest shape and outline and use of accessory muscles of respiration.

Come to terms: respiration

tachypnoea:	respiratory rate > 60 per minute
sternal retraction:	insuction of sternum in inspiration
intercostal recession:	excessive indrawing of intercostal muscles during respiration
periodic breathing:	alternating rhythm of respiration with periods of apnoea

Cardiovascular system

At the outset observe colour, respiratory effort, shape of chest, precordial bulge and/or heave. Localization of the trachea and the apex beat is important. The position of the apex beat may be difficult to localize but usually is between the 4th and 5th space in the midclavicular line. Precordial thrills are not uncommon in the neonate and should always be sought. Palpatation of the brachial and femoral pulse may require total concentration bearing in mind that too much pressure may obliterate it. The best advice is repetitive practice. The heart sounds should be listened to at both the apex and base commenting on the first sound at the apex and the second sound at the base. Not uncommonly a physiological third heart sound may be heard. The heart rate varies from 100 to 140 per minute. Occasionally extrasystoles may be noted and usually are of no significance. Heart block without a structural anomaly of the heart is extremely rare.

Systolic murmurs are common and usually best heard along the left sternal border. A short high pitched localized murmur which is not transmitted is generally benign and in the absence of any other positive finding a diagnosis of innocent murmur is made. As a precaution this should be rechecked before discharge and again at 3 and 6 weeks. The student should only be concerned with systolic murmurs in this age group. Listen to as many as possible — examine, examine, examine! When you improve and heart rate slows you may pick up diastolic murmurs.

Abdomen

Again, first observe. The abdomen is often generally somewhat distended — more so after a feed (so enquire!). Respiration is reflected in abdominal movement via the diaphragm and this is normal. If in doubt about distension measure at a marked point above or below the umbilicus. Observe the umbilicus. Is it ageing normally — any blood or discharges? Is there a smell, is there periumbilical inflammation, is the umbilical vein visible, is it inflammed? Reassure mother that the cord will part spontaneously around the fourth or fifth day. Is there any evidence of an early umbilical hernia? Occasionally palpation of the abdomen may cause the infant to regurgitate mucus or feed. So be careful.

Palpate the abdomen gently (with the aid of a soother if necessary). Use your right hand to examine for the spleen whose tip is often readily palpable. It does not matter what side you approach the examination of a newborn abdomen — just be comfortable. Check the liver edge by placing your palm between the umbilicus and right iliac crest. Get the feel of the abdomen and then slowly proceed towards the rib cage. Remember that the right lobe of the liver is what you are going to meet first. The liver edge is usually soft and easily missed. It is nearly always palpable up to 2–3 cm below the costal margin. There is little doubt that the kidneys in the average newborn can be palpated, particularly the lower poles. However, this is not easy and requires considerable practice. The most suitable method is to place one hand under the upper lumbar region exerting gentle pressure upwards whilst doing the actual palpation with the other hand. The examiner is trying to establish the presence of both kidneys and whether or not they are enlarged.

The bladder (when full) is an abdominal organ in the newborn and is best felt approximately 15 minutes after a feed. Starting just below the umbilicus using the index and second finger and thumb, gently feel for the bladder gradually moving pincer grasp downwards until felt. When a bladder is palpable gentle massage will produce a contraction following which a midstream specimen can be obtained without contamination. A large bladder is frequently noted where the infant is suffering from asphyxial encephalopathy or severe neural tube defect.

Note that inguinal lymph nodes are often palpable in the newborn and are a normal finding.

Genitalia

Female. Labia may be quite red and minora not covered particularly in the preterm. Labial fusion is sometimes present and is easily dealt with if required. Vaginal tags are common and should be ignored. They will resolve spontaneously during the first week. Vaginal haemorrhage ('newborn period') occasionally occurs. Bruising may be present particularly if the infant had a breech delivery. Increased pigmentation and enlargement of the clitoris should be noted.

Male. Is the penis of normal size and shape? Is there any evidence of hypospadias (epispadias is exceedingly rare)? Hypospadias is commonly glandular (or coronal), infrequently in the shaft (penile), and rarely at the base (perineal). Are the testes palpable and of normal size? If testes are not in the scrotum, commence in the inguinal area and palpate downwards. If a testis appears bigger than average, consider hydrocele (common) and confirm by transillumination. There may be an associated inguinal hernia which is more common in the male, particularly in the preterm. Very rarely an enlarged testis may be due to torsion; the testis then feels hard and is discoloured.

Musculo-skeletal system

The examination of bones, joints, ligaments and the attached muscles is of fundamental importance in the newborn.

Dislocatable (loose) hips

True dislocation is rare at birth with the notable exception of the infant with severe neural tube defect (meningomyelo-

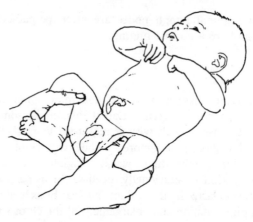

Fig. 4.2 Examining hips in the newborn infant.

cele). Unstable hip, however, is common and occurs in approximately 15–20 per 1000 live births. This condition is extremely uncommon in the preterm. Overall unstable hip is more common in the female except following breech presentation where the risk is equal in both sexes. Talipes calcaneo valgus may also be associated with it. The left hip is twice as likely to be involved than the right hip.

The earlier hip examination is carried out the better. Day one is now the day of choice with the best chance of positive diagnosis. In general, the Barlow method of examination is preferred. It is important that the infant is placed on a flat table (approximately waist high from the examiner), in the supine position and if possible relaxed. Position the hips and knees at 90° and grasp both knees between thumb and index and second fingers, the tips of which are over the outer trochanter of each femur. Press the hips gently backwards and then abduct and lift with the outside fingers — if the hip is loose a clunking feeling is noted when lifting the head of the femur back into the socket. The gentler this test is performed the better the response. It is very important to be gentle when carrying out this test and is certainly should not be done repetitively. It is very easy to damage the hip joint. Total abduction of the hip joint should never be carried out either during examination or treatment.

Feet

Mobility of the foot joints is the major factor determining the need for treatment or nontreatment. Deformities of the foot are common and vary in type.

Tarsus varus. This is extremely common — a degree occurs in nearly every infant. The foot is turned inwards to a varying degree at the tarsal joints. Spontaneous recovery is the rule though occasionally transient manipulation and massage may be necessary.

Calcaneo valgus. This condition is also common and appears to occur more often in the post term and may occasionally be associated with a loose hip. The dorsum of the foot is in position a close to the shin. As calf muscle tone improves the foot is pulled into the normal position; this usually occurs within 6 to 8 weeks.

Talipes equino varus (primary club foot). This condition occurs in 1 per 1000 births and is twice as common in the male infant. In 50% of cases it is bilateral. Usually there is a fixed structural deformity with involvement of both the fore and hindfoot and associated wasting of the calf muscles. Early manipulation and fixation is advisable.

Other minor anomalies of the toes occur including over-riding (usually 3rd or 4th) and overlapping of the 5th toe. Toenails always appear ingrowing in the newborn — this is a normal phenomenon. Therapy is usually not required for any of these conditions.

Minor *variants* not minor *anomalies*:
- mild to moderate bowing of lower leg
- mild syndactyly 2nd–3rd toes

- shallow sacral dimple
- hydrocele of testes
- single upper palmar crease.

Spine

Examination of the spinal processes should be carried out with the infant lying on one hand in the prone position and the other hand feeling the spine. Occasionally a spina bifida occulta or dermal sinus may be noted. More often a post anal dimple is present; this is of no consequence, and the mother should be reassured.

Central nervous system

Examination of this system in the newborn is entirely different from that of the older child. It is the assessment of posture and tone, movement and primitive reflexes. Therefore, much information may be obtained (once again) by spending a few minutes observing the infant. In general, the posture is entirely flexor though abnormal intrauterine posture can distort this, for example, extended breech or deflexed head. The complete flexor posture is not fully

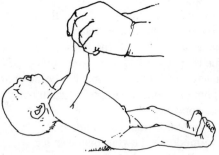

Fig. 4.3 Neck traction.

adopted until 37 completed weeks. Observe limb movements — are they normal? There is a great variation ranging from tremulous movements of one or all limbs to jittery movements, both of which may be normal. Feel the upper and lower limbs, establish flexor recoil and compare. If doubt exists then the examination should be repeated with the head held in the midline. Having the 'posture-picture' proceed to assess tone by doing the neck traction test. Here hands are firmly grasped and the infant is pulled to the sitting position. The head should flex and follow the traction to upright position and hold momentarily. This is an important test.

Vertical suspension is assessed by grasping the infant under each axilla. The normal infants supports himself in this position. The term infant who slips through is abnormal.

Ventral suspension is assessed by placing the infant prone on the palm of the hand. In the normal response the back extends, arms and knees flex, hips extend and head lifts and rotates.

Lower limb posture in the supine position is usually flexor with the hips slightly abducted. Full abduction of the hips in a supine term infant indicates hypotonia and is abnormal.

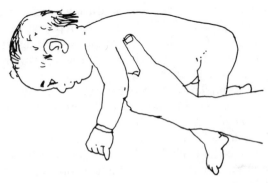

Fig. 4.4 Ventral suspension.

It must be stressed that when one or more of these tests suggest hypotonia a repeat examination in 24 hours may confirm or otherwise the significance of the previous examination. Remarkable changes in tone and posture can occur in a matter of hours during the first week of life.

Deep tendon reflexes can be readily elicited — particularly the knee tendon reflex. Flex the particular joint and hold the limb with the same hand and tap tendon with finger tip. Intermittent ankle clonus may also be present in the normal infant and is detected by gentle but sudden dosriflexion of the foot.

Pointers to hypotonia:
- head lag
- slips through on upright suspension
- like 'rag doll' in ventral suspension
- total hip abduction.

Primitive reflexes

A number of primitive reflexes are present and easily elicited in the normal term infant. These gradually disappear and are not present at the end of the sixth month with the notable exception of the blink response which remains. Do these tests properly since the best response is usually obtained on the first test. The response tends to wane on repeated testing.

Blink response. A gentle tap above the nasal bridge usually evokes the blink response. This test is nearly always normal except in the very ill infant.

Cardinal signs. These collectively refer to sensory stimulation of the cheek and skin around the mouth and lips. Pressing a finger on the cheek near the mouth and moving it latterly will cause the infant to open his mouth and turn the head to root for a nipple. When a finger, soother or nipple is placed in the mouth, the normal infant will suck vigorously (depending somewhat on the timing of the previous feed) and swallow in unison.

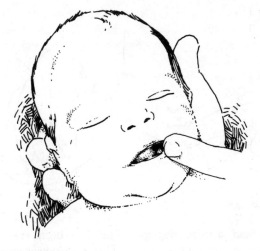

Fig. 4.5 Cardinal points.

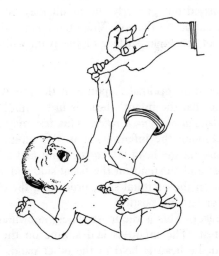

Fig. 4.6 Palmar grasp.

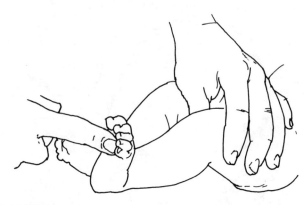

Fig. 4.7 Toe grasp.

Grasp and traction response. This has been referred to previously in relation to tone. This test however can be provoked unilaterally by placing a finger or pencil in the infants plam. This causes grasping and with gentle upward traction the forearm and shoulder muscles will contract. When carried out properly the infant may be lifted 2–3 cm from the surface of the cot. When the infant is lowered gentle stroking of the ulnar surface of the palm will disengage the grasp.

To record an optimal response in the following tests it is preferable that the infant's head is in the midline.

Asymmetrical tonic neck reflex. This test may easily be elicited by leaving the infant lying in the supine position and slowly turning the head 90° to the right and left. The upper and lower limbs extend on the facial side and similarly there is flexion on the occipital side, producing the classical sword fighting or fencing posture.

Moro reflex. This is the most widely known and frequently elicited test. The infant is laid supine on the forearm and hand and the head is held in the other hand. The response

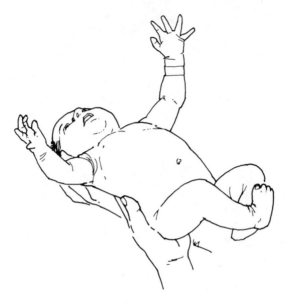

Fig. 4.8 Moro response.

occurs when the head is 'dropped' a few centimetres. The upper limbs abduct, extend and flex in a flowing movement symmetrically. A poor or no response indicates a major problem. However, a unilateral response confirms the damage (usually transient) to the 5th and 6th cervical roots producing the classical Erb's paresis.

Spinal curve or Galant reflex. Hold the infant on one hand (similar to ventral suspension test) and stroke the lateral border of the spinal muscle from the midthoracic area downwards. This will cause the pelvis to curve to the same side. A similar response should be evoked on the opposite side.

Crossed extension reflex. While keeping the infant in the supine position, extend one knee and stroke the foot on the same side, this will cause the opposite leg to flex, abduct and extend 'to push away' the provoking hand.

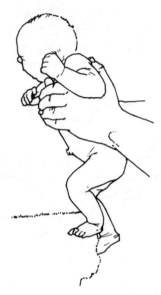

Fig. 4.9 Placing reflex.

Extensor thrust, placing and walking reflex. These movements relate and provide evidence of lower limb function. With the infant held between both hands, the legs lowered to the surface and pressure on the soles of the feet may cause the lower limbs to suddenly extend producing an extensor thrust. If the lower limbs, with the infant still held in the same position, are pressed against the edge of examining table one foot will flex to place. By bringing the infant's limbs further on to the table leaning forwards at an angle of 10–20° a walking movement may be produced.

Hearing. A crude hearing response can certainly be elicited in the newborn. The simplest test is to say 'aaah' into the crying infant's ear from a distance of 3–4 cm. Usually this produces a cessation of crying. A startle response to a loud noise may be a crude indicator of hearing.

Vision. The newborn can see and will readily turn to a light source. The infant may, for example, turn his head to the room or cubicle window. Also when seated comfortably and with the infant held in the supine facing the examiner at an angle of about 30°, eye fixation can be established at a distance of about 20 cm. A red ball of 5–6 cm in diameter can be brought slowly across the infants visual field at which time following may occur. These latter tests require time, a cooperative infant, and certain expertise. Positive responses to vision and hearing tests are very reassuring to the mother.

Newborn examination: purposes

Day 1:	1. To assess general condition
	2. To establish normality
	3. To detect major abnormalities
Day 3–5:	1. To confirm normality
(discharge)	2. To detect minor abnormalities
	3. To assess neurological status

Conclusion

Examination of the central nervous system in the newborn requires attention to detail, a deal of patience and a baby in the right mood. The value of transient alteration of one, two or even three tests is as yet not precisely clear. However, much research has and is being carried out in this area and there is little doubt that diligent and repetitive examination can be both rewarding and educational. The record of such a detailed examination may be of vital importance to the developmental paediatrician in later years.

SIX WEEKS EXAMINATION

The six weeks examination is an important postnatal event and *all* babies should be seen at this time.

The purposes of the six week examination are:
- to evaluate feeding pattern
- to measure growth and weight gain
- to detect abnormalities not noted in neonatal period
- to assess early development
- to ensure infant-maternal bonding.

It is important at six weeks assessment to have all the relevant perinatal details including birthweight, head circumference and crown heel length.

Measurement (centiles):
- Head circumference
- Length
- Weight.

Adverse perinatal history to note:
- asphyxia
- low birthweight
- infection
- hypoglycaemia
- trauma.

The process of examination should be careful and gentle. Take the fully dressed infant from his mother and lay him on a covered table. You should not allow the mother or nurse or anyone else to undress the infant. Do it yourself as the examination proceeds, get the feel of the baby yourself. Observe, without disturbing if possible. Look at the way the infant is dressed and the general picture of care. Look at the face — good colour, clean, no rash, scalp clear, normal quiet respiration or otherwise, any evidence of snuffles or noisy breathing? Is there any evidence of anaemia? Are the lips a good colour? Gently check the conjunctiva.

Feel the head and fontanelle, look for seborrhoea. If the infant is awake, try and get eye fixation from about 20 cm. Having achieved eye fixation often the baby will smile in return. *Smiling with meaning is an important milestone.* If however, the infant is crying say 'aaah' into his ear in low tone and crying may cease. If it does not, hold the infant upright and tip him forwards. Crying may cease and eyes open. Then start again.

Now check head growth, feel anterior fontanelle and sutures. Look for early head control. When holding the infant in the sitting position the head should fall forward and there should be reasonable, if wobbly head control. Look at limb movements and check limb tone. Observe the hands — look for thumb abduction and finger flexion. If fisting is present open the palm, observe for accumulation of dirt in the palmar creases. The skin of the palm may be moist and pale. This suggests the hands have been tightly clenched since birth. Look for persistent ankle clonus. Check primitive reflexes, looking for accentuation of particularly the Moro, asymmetrical tonic neck and walking reflexes. Now proceed to undress the infant yourself — leave the nappy on (for obvious reasons) for the moment and look at the state of nutrition, respiratory rate, general well-being. Is there any evidence of dehydration, loss of subcutaneous fat or wasting. Gently examine mouth, particularly observing for evidence of monilial infection. Look for evidence of conjunctival infection. Roll tip of finger over inner canthus to clear lacrimal duct.

Developmental indicators:

- frowning: 3–6 weeks
- smiling with meaning: 5–8 weeks
- early head control (5–10 sec):   5–8 weeks

- eye fixation on examination of face: 6 weeks
                                          (20–30 cm)
- vocalization (coo) may be present: 6 weeks
        (usually in an infant with siblings).

Transient blockage of nasolacrimal duct is very common. Check nose for snuffles — again an extremely common finding and usually of no serious consequence. Swelling of the infant's breasts may be present, and occasionally there is evidence of inflammation and abscess formation. Inflammation and infection of the corners of the finger and toenails (paronychia) are fairly common.

Skin

Look for evidence of seborrhoea in the scalp and/or napkin dermatitis. Usually facial 'stork bite marks' are fading. Conversely strawberry naevi have become more defined and are growing. Port wine stain unfortunately has become more defined as the skin becomes paler. Occasionally physiological jaundice may have persisted in association with breast milk feeding. However, the re-emergence of jaundice at 6 weeks is a sinister sign and must be thoroughly investigated.

Respiratory

Observe the infant's rate and type of breathing. Is it noisy? If so, what kind of noise — upper, lower, inspiratory or expiratory? Laryngomalacia is a common cause of inspiratory stridor in this age group. Coughing implies a lower respiratory infection — though specific abnormal sounds are rarely localized on auscultation.

CVS

Heart rate and pulses should be checked. The pulse will alter significantly if crying. Check the precordium and apex beat. Remember a thrill is more easily felt in this age-group. Listen to the heart sounds at the apex and also at the base, commenting on the first sound in the former and the second sound at the latter. Is there a murmur, which, with few notable exceptions, is nearly always systolic in nature? Where is it best localized — does it radiate, is it loud, is there a thrill and more important of all, what is the duration, is it pansystolic? Try to decide if the murmur is significant or not.

Remember — a benign systolic murmur is short, high pitched, soft, not transmitted and there is no thrill. A venous hum (more common in toddlers) may be heard at the base. Pressure in the jugular vein should reduce this sound considerably.

Abdomen

Look at the shape. Is there any distension, has the umbilicus healed completely, is there any residual granulation tissue or is there any herniation? Palpate for the spleen, the tip of which may well be palpable. Feel the liver edge (2–3 cm) and percuss if necessary. Check for palpable bladder and perhaps lower poles of kidney. This latter examination becomes more difficult as the infants get older. Look at the genitalia. Are both testes palpable? Is there any evidence of hydrocele or inguinal hernia? Is there a reasonable prepucial opening? In the female, check for labial fusion. Look at the anus, observe for blood staining and/or early fissure — a not uncommon problem.

Musculo-skeletal

In the majority the feet are normal, tarsus varus and calcaneus valgus having resolved spontaneously in the previous 4 weeks.

Examination of the hips is again important though much less rewarding than during the first week. Again use Barlow test. One may find benign adductor spasm in some infants. Do not force the hips into full abduction as this manoeuvre can damage the hip joint. Subluxation at 6 weeks is rare.

3 Hs to highlight at 6 weeks

1. Head: too big = ? hydrocephalus
                too small = ? microcephaly
2. Heart: murmurs may become apparent!
3. Hips: last chance to detect CHD before walking?

A thorough examination is from head to toe and is easy to do. 6-week-old babies and their mothers usually enjoy this examination.

Warning signals: 6 weeks

- major maternal anxiety
- unusually small or large head
- *hypotonia* = poor ventral suspension
                 poor neck traction
- persistent irritability
- persistent thumb adduction.

THE ACUTELY ILL INFANT

It is clear that further improvements in infant mortality will require doctors to sharpen their diagnostic wits and instincts. Infants have a very limited clinical vocabulary with which to express themselves and the identical symptoms (food refusal, vomiting, fever, lethargy) may reflect meningitis, pneumonia, or urinary tract infection.

Infants can become ill very rapidly — happily for the practising doctor they also recover promptly if appropriately treated. In infancy one must always heed the mother's judgement and opinion. We will not repeat the importance in approaching ill infants of:

- careful observation
- thorough examination
- instinctual suspicion.

Certain symptoms in infancy demand our immediate attention. Below are listed some of them. Mothers will vary in their rapidity of response but most will recognize the seriousness of these complaints and seek help. Mothers in our country use the idiomatic expression 'he's not himself' to imply a significant change in their infant's well-being.

Always serious symptoms in infancy:
- high pitched screaming or crying
- alternating drowsiness and irritability
- convulsion
- refusal to feed (two or more consecutive feeds)
- repeated vomiting
- rapid, laboured breathing, with or without grunting
- episodes of unusual blueness or paleness.

A quotation from an old Dublin textbook of children's diseases seems pertinent: 'the child when ill is more or less peevish — dislikes being stirred or even cries when being handled; its hour of sleep is uncertain and it rests ill, or awakes startled and crying . . . when a sick child is brought to us or we visit it, our attention should be first directed to the expression of the countenance, then to the attitude, state of the limbs, and skin' (Evanson & Maunsell 1840 *A practical treatise on the management and diseases of children.* Fannin, Dublin). How true and well said. The sick child lies down and does not want to be disturbed. He'll get up if and when he's better.

The acutely ill infant (especially with meningitis) does not like being handled, resents disturbance, and sleeps more than usual. When awake he may be restless, irritable and difficult to placate. Maternal expressions for this state include 'grizzly', 'cranky', and 'wingeing'.

Less serious symptoms, but ones not to be ignored are detailed below. Infants with these complaints will need to be kept under close observation. Croup is a source of great parental anxiety even though their infant may be apparently coping.

Usually serious symptoms in infancy:

- repeated diarrhoea
- prolonged crying
- croup (stridor, hoarseness, barking cough)
- high fever (40°C–104°F)
- persistent crankiness.

One's first approach to the acutely and seriously ill infant is to observe the infant in his position of comfort. Note the heart rate, respiratory rate and effort, presence or absence of a rash, colour and temperature. Ill infants frequently have a mottled (or marbled) appearance to their skin. They lie still. Breathing is often rapid and grunting. The eyes have a glazed or distant look. They may be centrally warm and peripherally cold. They convulse easily with fever.

Note movement (or lack of it). Refusal to use a limb may suggest infection therein, for example, osteomyelitis. Splinting of the chest is occasionally seen in pneumonia. Arching of the neck occurs with meningitis. An immobile abdomen is very significant, appendicitis and peritonitis being notoriously difficult to detect in infancy.

One needs to make a statement about:

- degree of sickness
- hydration
- nutrition
- circulation.

Before proceeding to detailed examination, weight, temperature pulse rate, respiratory rate will of course be recorded. Ill infants are usually fairly passive and can be examined in an organized fashion.

Degree of sickness

This can only be learned and not taught in texts or tutorials.

So do spend time in the emergency room and admitting office. See and assess, regard and remember. Is he seriously ill? Is he moderately ill? Is he mildly ill?

Hydration

This can easily and rapidly be assessed (see p. 152). One wishes to determine if the infant is normally hydrated, dehydrated, or less commonly, over hydrated.

Nutrition

Nutrition can be quickly assessed by looking and feeling subcutaneous fat, inspecting buttocks and muscle bulk, looking for lax skinfolds in the axilla and groin, and of course weighing the infant. Skinfold thickness and mid arm circumference can be determined later if necessary. Is he plump, 'normal', or poorly nourished?

Circulation

What is his circulation like? Is the colour of tongue, lips, mucous membranes and nail beds normal? Is he mottled or cyanosed? Are the peripheries warm? Is venous filling in the feet reasonably rapid? Warm toes (especially with palpable

Acute illness in infancy

Medical sickness	Surgical sickness
Meningitis	Intussusception
Pneumonia	Appendicitis/peritonitis
Osteomyelitis	Intestinal obstruction
Gastroenteritis	Incarcerated hernia
Septicaemia	
Urinary tract infection	
Croup syndromes	

dorsalis pedis or posterior tibial pulses) are a reasonably good indicator of satisfactory circulatory state. One must not omit to measure blood pressure in acutely ill infants.

Simply by *looking* at a baby or infant you can make some useful statements as for example:

- normal infant
- moderately ill
- normally hydrated
- well nourished
- possibly anaemic
- query respiratory tract infection.

Food refusal is a serious symptom in infancy. By contrast, the infant who feeds well may be ill, but not seriously so. We reassure mothers that their infants are reasonably well if they fulfill the 3 Fs:

- good *form*
- good *feeding*
- no *fever*.

THE TERRIFIED TODDLER

That enfant terrible of paediatrics, the toddler (1–3 years) warrants special mention. He can be clinging, resistive, screaming or downright impossible to examine. Approach him as you would any creature who feels he is cornered — slowly, carefully and with calculated caution. With experience and expertise you may be able to examine him surreptitiously and superficially. Do not remove him from his place of safety, his mother's knee, or embrace. He does not like having his head circumference measured, his ear drums examined or his throat inspected; leave these till last. Give him toys (or even spatulae) to occupy both hands. Above all learn to be expedient and speedy in your examination. But don't rush him. The simple ploy of first placing your stethoscope on his knee may enable him to allow you to auscultate his heart.

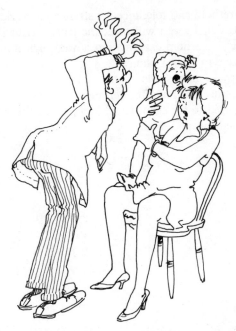

Fig. 4.10 The terrified toddler.

One will always have to use one's wits and instincts in approaching the toddler. A lot can be achieved by examining him when asleep — you can observe colour, note rate and depth of respiration, palpate the pulse (e.g. pre-auricular), feel his skin temperature, see if he's coping and comfortable, determine hydration and nutrition, and assess circulation (by feeling toe temperature). Diagnosis by eye and by instinct. The experienced observer can quickly decide whether the sleeping toddler is seriously ill or not.

Some toddlers defy proper examination despite stealth and patience. Try again when he may be in more benign humour. John Apley (a famous paediatrician) has said 'It's my fault if a child cries'. We would not entirely agree. Toddlers have a very low threshold and tolerance for strange faces and stethoscopes. Occasionally you will meet the truly terrified toddler (a 'screamer') on whom examination is well nigh impossible. One may have to record failure:

fundoscopy — impossible

blood pressure not recorded (crying)

and be prepared to try again later. Some 'tricks of the trade' are mentioned, on p. 175.

5

Systems examination

THE CHEST

The single most common reason for infants and toddlers to present to their family doctor is an acute respiratory tract infection, usually upper (see Ear, nose, mouth and throat). However, the good observer can often distinguish between infections involving the upper and/or lower respiratory tract by looking and listening carefully. All too often students are keen to get their hands and stethoscopes into play. Better to stand back and observe.

Observe the pattern of breathing, the work of breathing, the rate of breathing. Listen for an expiratory grunt. Note the type of cough. Does the infant display frothiness or flaring of the alae nasi? Does he have a wheeze? Can he cope with a feed? What is his colour like?

History

The history in respiratory tract infection consists of some combination or permutation of the symptoms of cough, wheeze, stridor, croup, poor feeding and fever. In more severe cases there may be rapid respiration, grunting, cyanosis, restlessness or even collapse.

It is very difficult to individually distinguish viral from

bacterial infections. However we have found 'Lightwood's law' to be of some value: this states that bacterial infections tend to localize — to one ear, to a tonsil, to a lobe of lung, whereas viral infections tend to spread. Measles is a good example of a spreading virus — red eyes, red ears, red throat, red skin and, if you could see it, red trachea. 'Toxicity' is difficult to clinically describe. Children with severe bacterial infections tend to be more 'toxic' — more sick, more still, more mottled.

It is also useful to try to distinguish upper from lower respiratory infections, remembering that URTI and LRTI can co-exist.

One should attempt to correctly sequence from the onset of symptoms, as for example:

cough for 4 days
poor feeding for 2 days
fever for 2 days
wheeze for 1 day
dyspnoea for 1 day.

It may be important to ask:

Which came first, the cough or the wheeze?
Is he getting progressively worse?
Has he maintained a good colour?
Can he manage a bottle or feed?

The four components of examination of the respiratory system are inspection, palpation, percussion and auscultation. Of these *inspection* is surely the most valuable, especially in infants. By inspection we include listening as well as looking. We find ourselves frequently reminding students that the experienced paediatric ward sister can make an accurate stab at diagnosis from the door of the cubicle nursing an infant with an acute respiratory infection.

Palpation and percussion are not particularly useful exercises in acute LRTI's in infants and toddlers. The liver is frequently pushed down by a flattened diaphragm, the trachea is rarely displaced and demonstration of hepatic or cardiac dullness not particularly helpful. Lobar pneumonias demonstrable as dullness to percussion are infrequent in infancy. It must be emphasized that the above remarks are applicable only to infants. In childhood the traditional arts of percussion and palpation, as taught in 'adult' medicine are important.

Inspection

Inspection will include comments on and recording:

1. Colour.
2. How the child is coping: Is he comfortable? Is he noisy but managing? Is he in respiratory distress? Is he unstable, with very laboured breathing?
3. What is his position of comfort?
4. Respiratory rate — what is normal for a given age (see below)?
5. Chest movement. Is it symmetrical? Is there splinting of one side of the chest?
6. Chest shape. Is the chest overblown or barrel shaped? Is there pectus excavatum (hollow chest), pectus carinatum (pigeon chest) or Harrison's sulcus?
7. Pursing of lips in expiration?
8. Presence of frothiness, nasal flaring or grunting?
9. Type of respiratory movement. Normal respiration is a quiet in-out movement of the chest.
10. Dyspnoea? This will be manifest by increased respiratory effort 'at rest'. Increased work of respiration is shown by suprasternal, intercostal and subcostal recession. Unilateral recession is sometimes seen in lobar pneumonia or with inhaled foreign body.

Come to terms: breathing

tachypnoea	= increased rate of respiration
dyspnoea	= laboured or difficult respiration
hyperpnoea (hyperventilation)	= increased depth of respiration
orthopnoea	= dyspnoea at rest

Normal respiratory rate (at rest)

Age	Range of normal (resps/min)	Rapid
Newborn	30–50	> 60
Infancy	20–30	> 50
Toddler	20–30	> 40
Children	15–20	> 30

11. Is there finger clubbing? Clubbing of fingers and toes in children is usually secondary to cyanotic congenital heart disease or to chronic suppurative lung disease. If unsure about finger clubbing, look at the great toe. Clubbing may also

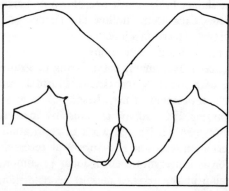

Fig. 5.1 Schramroth's sign.

be familial or associated with chronic diarrhoeal states. You may find Schramroth's sign helpful. Normal fingers have a 'window' between opposed nails; clubbed fingers have no window and an increased angle.

Come to terms: chest shapes

pectus carinatum	= prominent sternum; pigeon breast
pectus excavatum	= marked sternal depression
Harrison's sulcus	= indrawing of lower chest with rib flaring (diaphragmatic tug)

12. Presence of sputum: the expectoration of sputum is a relative rarity in young children, being mainly the province of children with chronic suppurative lung disease, for example cystic fibrosis. Even though a cough may correctly be called productive in infancy, sputum is not seen since it is swallowed. Evanson & Maunsell (1838) correctly stated 'the young child almost always swallows any matter expectorated, and therefore this can scarcely become an object of diagnosis'. The swallowing of sputum is partly responsible for the vomiting which frequently follows a bout of coughing in childhood. Post-tussive vomiting is most typically seen in pertussis.

13. Traumatic petechiae may sometimes be seen on the eyelids, face and around the neck following a severe bout of coughing. They may also occur following prolonged crying or enforced restraint as for a lumbar puncture.

Palpation should include a comment on symmetry and extent of chest expansion. Chest expansion should be about 3–5 cms in school age children.

The position of the trachea should be determined. Deviation of the trachea is infrequent in infants and toddlers.

Vocal fremitus can be assessed by palpation of the infant's chest when crying. Transmitted sounds may be palpated.

Percussion should of course be performed gently, comparing sides. The percussion note in infants and toddlers tends to be more resonant than in adults. Detailed percussion in infants and toddlers may not be very rewarding. However, in the preschool and schoolchild percussion should be carried out as in the adult.

Asthma at first sight?

Asthmatic children may have:

- jerky respiration (up-down chest movement rather than in-out movement)
- a tendency to raise their shoulders towards their ears on deep inspiration
- an overblown upper chest while the lower chest may have an early Harrison's sulcus.

Auscultation

The stethoscope

The stethoscope should preferably have a paediatric diaphragm and bell; one sees many students today using the diaphragm for all purposes. The bell is a much more useful sound-piece for infants, toddlers and children.

The bell is best

- the bell is smaller — the diaphragm of an adult stethoscope covers a large area of the chest of a neonate or infant
- the bell is warmer — diaphragms can be very cold
- the bell applies better to the chest

- the bell allows less surface noise and is better attuned to receive low pitched chest sounds. Indeed, the latterday chest physician had no diaphragm on his stethoscope. Widespread use of the diaphragm for auscultating chests is undesirable and deplorable. The diaphragm is primarily designed for cardiac signs and sounds.

Auscultation implies use of the ear plus the stethoscope. Always listen carefully to the type of cough and attempt to describe it carefully. Listen for a grunt. An expiratory grunt is very suggestive of a pneumonic process. An audible wheeze, usually expiratory is heard in a wide variety of childhood lower respiratory infections, from wheezy bronchitis to bronchiolitis to bronchopneumonia. An expiratory wheeze with prolonged expiratory phase is very typical of bronchospasm associated with acute asthma.

It is important to remember that the stethoscope can be an unreliable instrument in the infant. One is occasionally struck by the finding of pneumonia on chest radiograph in an infant whose chest seemed remarkably clear.

A few words on transmitted sounds. These are often heard in infants, especially frothy mucousy infants and can cause confusion for students. Transmitted sounds are sounds transmitted from the oropharynx to the chest, and are common in infants and toddlers. These noises arise from secretions in the upper respiratory tract especially the oropharynx. Suction, coughing and physiotherapy may clear such sounds. They are rough, sometimes leathery sounds often mistaken by students for a pleural rub at first hearing.

The thinwalled infant's chest wall allows easy conduction of sound from one side to another and gives the impression of increased intensity of breath sounds to the unfamiliar ear. Breath sounds in infancy have a bronchovesicular character. In the preschool and schoolchild breath sounds assume the familiar vesicular quality heard in the adult.

One needs to develop the ability to listen between cries, to ignore surface movements and transmitted sounds and to compare intensity of breath sounds from side to side.

Pleural rub is an infrequent finding in preschool children.

Adventitious sounds

Wheeze = rhonchus = continuous sound = dry sound.
Crackle = crepitation = discontinuous sound = wet sound.

Wheeze in infants is due to air movement through a narrowed airway, the narrowing of the tube being caused by

1. mucosal oedema
2. excessive mucus
3. bronchospasm.

Of these bronchospasm is probably the least important. Several studies have failed to show any appreciable effects of bronchodilators on wheezy infants less than 1 year of age. We can all see the 'runny nose' of rhinitis; consider the 'runny chest' as analagous. Wheeze can occur in a variety of chest infections, as shown below.

Wheeze associated respiratory infections (WARI)

- acute laryngotracheobronchitis
- acute bronchitis
- acute bronchiolitis
- acute bronchopneumonia.

There is lack of unformity and consistency in the terminology of acute bronchitis. We accept the terms wheezy bronchitis and spasmodic bronchitis as synonymous. Winter bronchitis is not a helpful term. Most infants who wheeze in infancy wheeze infrequently and with infection. When wheeze is recurrent the correct term is usually asthma, or if you wish, asthmatic bronchitis. There are, of course, other causes of recurrent wheeze including aspiration syndromes, foreign body, cystic fibrosis and tracheal compression.

A useful exercise in many systems, including the respiratory system, is to draw out one's findings in diagrammatic form. Some examples are shown in Figures 5.2 and 5.3.

Rhonchi (wheeze, dry sounds) and crepitations (crackles, rales, wet sounds) are no different in children than in adults and we will not describe them. However, it is wise to remember that rhonchi in infants are generated by air flow through a tube narrowed by oedema and mucus rather than to bronchospasm per se.

In approaching diagnosis in respiratory infection we find it useful to divide the respiratory tract into upper, middle and lower. One too often meets the lazy diagnosis 'URTI' or 'chest infection' in charts today. This represents clinical vagueness and uncertainty. One should attempt to be more specific. There are at least six URTI's and 'chest infections'.

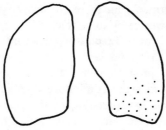

Fig. 5.2 Left basal crepitations.

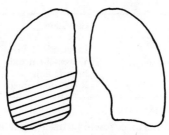

Fig. 5.3 Right middle and lower lobe consolidation.

In a similar vein, the modern term 'pneumonitis' is equally imprecise.

URTI: **upper respiratory tract infection**

rhinitis	otitis	sinusitis
tonsillitis	mastoiditis	pharyngitis

The term 'croup' has come to be a diagnosis. It is not.

The word croup, from the Scottish word 'croak' describes the harsh, crowing, vibratory inspiratory stridor, usually accompanied by a barking croup and hoarseness. Croup has many causes including infection, allergy and foreign body.

Croup: middle respiratory tract infection
            spasmodic laryngitis
            laryngotracheobronchitis LTB
            epiglottitis.

Similarly, the diagnostic designation of 'chest infection' is not worthy of a medical student or doctor. 'Chest infection' is a layman's term. Again there are many types of infection involving the lower respiratory tract.

LRTI: **lower respiratory tract infection**

tracheitis	pneumonia	bronchiolitis
bronchitis	bronchopneumonia	empyema.

While diagnosis in acute respiratory tract infection rests on a summation and interpretation of the findings, experience has taught us that certain signs in infancy are highly suspicious of certain conditions. Some examples are listed below:

Sign	Condition
Croup	Laryngitis, LTB
Wheeze	Wheezy bronchitis
Full chest, frothiness	Bronchiolitis
Flaring, grunting	Bronchopneumonia

Somebody has described *grunting* as a form of 'auto-PEEP' (that is, automatic positive end-expiratory pressure).

Occasional chest findings

1. *Pleuritic pain*: children with pneumonia do occasionally complain of sharp, severe pleuritic pain. Those old enough will point to the area. Younger children may 'splint' the affected side. In our experience a pleural rub is a rare finding in childhood, particularly in preschool children.
2. *Pneumothorax*: a small pneumothorax or pneumomediastum may occasionally complicate acute asthma or a severe coughing spell in childhood (for example with pertussis). The pneumothorax is not usually clinically demonstrable; however auscultation of a loud crunching noise synchronous with cardiac systole is characteristic.
3. *Subcutaneous emphysema*: is sometimes seen in acute asthma. The cardinal clinical sign is a crackling feeling over the upper anterior chest, over the clavicles or in the neck.
4. Children with asthma sometimes complain of an *itch* in their throat.

Wheezy bronchitis

Symptoms	Signs
Cough	
Wheeze	Tachypnoea, recession
Low grade fever	Audible wheeze
Variable upset	Bilateral rhonchi

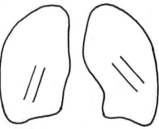

Fig. 5.4 Wheezy bronchitis.

Bronchiolitis

Symptoms	Signs
Cough	Oral frothiness
Wheeze	Respiratory difficulty
Rapid breathing	Overinflated chest
	Diffuse crepitations
Poor feeding	Bilateral rhonchi

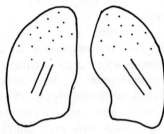

Fig. 5.5 Bronchiolitis.

Bronchopneumonia

Symptoms	Signs
Cough	Flaring of alae nasi
Wheeze	Grunting
Irritability	Respiratory difficulty
Fever	Unilateral or bilateral crepitations
Poor feeding	Occasional rhonchi

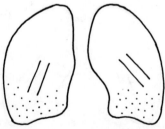

Fig. 5.6 Bronchopneumonia.

Textbooks tend to try to classify and may by times over-simplify. Bronchiolitis and bronchopneumonia can in practice be difficult to distinguish, the balance being tipped one way or the other, perhaps, by chest radiograph or peripheral white cell count.

A compendium of coughs

Cough may be dry or moist (productive). A productive cough results from an inflammatory or infective exudate on the bronchial mucosa. An intermittent or persistent dry cough may imply irritation of the upper respiratory tract or of the bronchial wall by a foreign body or extrinsic mass (glands). The appearance and amount of sputum should be assessed, remembering that children under 5 years swallow sputum. Clear, mucoid sputum or tacky tenacious sputum are often indicative of asthma. Green, yellow, grey ('dirty') sputum usually indicate the presence of infection. Haemoptysis is now a rare phenomenon in children of developed countries, other than in children with advanced cystic fibrosis.

Listen to coughs and try to describe them. Below are listed some of the commoner varieties.

- croupy cough: barking associated with stridor and hoarseness

Type and timing of cough

Cough	Suggests
Non productive nocturnal	Post nasal drip, asthma
On exercise	Asthma
Paroxysmal	Pertussis, foreign body
During or after feed	Inhalation
Productive in morning	Cystic fibrosis, asthma
Bovine, brassy	Tracheitis
Absence during sleep	Psychogenic

- whooping cough: inspiratory gasp, prolonged distressing cough, ending in a whoop, followed by vomiting
- 'chesty' cough: moist, fruity productive cough.

The type and timing of a cough can be important in deciding on the underlying respiratory problem.

THE CARDIOVASCULAR SYSTEM

Congenital heart disorders, with an incidence of close to 1 per 100 newborn infants, are the second most common defects encountered. About half of congenital heart disorders may be detected in the neonatal period; the remaining cases will not present until later — hence the importance of routine examination at various ages. There are some 40 described varieties of congenital heart disorders (CHD), of which only about 10 are frequent. For convenience we might classify them as follows:

Cyanotic CHD-: transposition of the great vessels
Fallot's tetralogy
pulmonary atresia

Potentially cyanotic CHD-(left-right shunts): atrial septal defect
ventricular septal defect
patent ductus arteriosus

Obstructive CHD- : coarctation of aorta
pulmonary stenosis
aortic stenosis

The *symptoms* and *signs* suggesting congestive cardiac failure associated with congenital heart disease in infancy are:

1. Tachypnoea (respiratory rare > 50–60 at rest).

2. Dyspnoea at rest or following a feed. Inability to finish a feed due to dyspnoea is characteristic.

3. Sweating. Some refer to the circle of sweat on the sheet around the infant's head as the 'halo sign'.

4. Unusual weight gain, greater than expected for caloric intake.

5. Tachycardia (heart rate > 140–160 at rest).

6. Hepatomegaly.

7. Gallop rhythm.

8. Cyanosis, especially central. Nursing the infant in 100% oxygen may help to distinguish cardiac from respiratory cyanosis.

Note that pulmonary crepitations and oedema are relatively late signs of cardiac failure.

Approach to cardiovascular examination

Start at the periphery and work towards the heart. Look for cyanosis, clubbing, respiratory difficulty, anaemia or polycythaemia. Jugular venous pulse and pressure are difficult to appreciate in infancy due to the relative shortness of the neck.

We would agree with John Apley's approach to examination of the heart: 'use your eyes and hands before your ears. Leave the heart to last; and when you come to it leave auscultation to the last'.

The pulse

Pulses should be felt over the radial, brachial and femoral arteries. Preferably use finger pulps; if in difficulty use of thumbs is allowable, if not desirable. Femoral pulses, often difficult to palpate, must always be sought, otherwise coarctation of the aorta will be missed. If femoral pulses are thought to be diminished, look for evidence of radio-femoral delay — this can be hard to detect at rapid heart rates.

Palpation of the dorsalis pedis pulse effectively excludes coarctation in infancy. Preauricular pulse is easily felt in sleeping infants.

Pulse volume

Is the pulse of normal, full or small volume? Appreciation of normal volume, with the finger pulp or tips implies palpation of many pulses. Full volume pulses, due to a wide pulse pressure, are best appreciated at the radial pulse; easily palpable foot pulses in neonates and infants may be indicative of increased pulse pressure.

A thready, weak or small volume pulse is indicative of reduced pulse pressure. Most often it is felt in hypotension or impending shock in infants. Pulsus paradoxus is an appreciable change in pulse volume with respiration.

Pulse rate

Pulse rate is related to age and activity with variations brought on by distress, fever, excitement and exercise. The value of simple but careful observation of the pulse can be emphasized by the fact that the earliest signs of rheumatic fever are (a) a fixed tachycardia (no variation, between sleep and awake pulse) and (b) loss of sinus arrhythmia.

The pulse rate will rise approximately 10 per minute for every 1°C rise in temperature.

Normal heart rate at rest

Age	Average rate	Upper limit of normal
0–6 months	140	160
6–12 months	130	150
1–2 years	110	130
2–6 years	100	120
6–10 years	95	110
10–14 years	85	100

Normal pulse variation

- sinus arrythmia — an increase in pulse rate on inspiration, with slowing on expiration. Very common in children
- occasional ectopics — need be of no concern
- bradycardia (pulse rate < 60) in fit children and adolescents, especially in good swimmers
- slight tachycardia with excitement due, for example, to clinic attendance or hospital admission

Blood pressure

Is dealt with on p. 82. Postural hypotension is an infrequent finding in children. Appreciation of postural hypotension (a fall of 20 mm systolic blood pressure on adopting the upright posture) is an important sign of hypovolaemia.

Blood pressure should be routinely measured in infants and children with congenital heart disease. Indeed we suggest BP measurement on all children admitted to hospital, on most attending outpatient clinics, and in all sick infants and neonates.

Colour

Central cyanosis is easily detected. Prolonged central cyanosis may result in plethoric appearance due to polycythaemia. Children with severe cyanosis sometimes adopt the squatting position after exercise — this increases peripheral resistance, increases pulmonary venous return and increases left to right shunting of blood.

Clubbing is dealt with on p. 68

Blood pressure

The most obvious statement about children's blood pressure

is that it is not taken. Not taken at all, not taken often enough, or not taken seriously. It is too often held that measurement of blood pressure in infants and children is difficult and time-consuming, and usually normal. Measurement of blood pressure in children merely requires patience, practice and a selection of cuffs from 3–13 cm wide.

Technique

Record blood pressure on right arm.

Child preferably seated or standing.

Child should be relaxed — pressures recorded during crying are unreliable.

Use the largest cuff width which comfortably fits the upper arm.

Ensure the inner bladder encircles the arm.

Doppler ultrasound recording for neonates and infants.

Standard auscultatory sphygmomanometry for older children.

Keep arm — heart — sphygmomanometer on same horizontal plane.

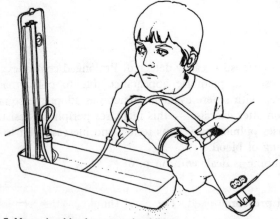

Fig. 5.7 Measuring blood pressure in children.

Diastolic pressure preferably recorded at point of disappearance (phase 4).

If there is significant difference between Phase 4 (muffling) and Phase 5 (disappearance of sounds), record both points.

Suggested shorthand notation for BP:

    ♀̣ standing

    Ⴑ sitting

   o—< lying

Note arm used and cuff size.

Remember that anxiety plus faulty technique are probably the commonest explanations of elevated blood pressure in children. Single raised values are of no significance; they must be repeated several times. Blood pressures recorded on admission to hospital are notoriously unreliable. The combination of anxiety plus obesity in the child may also falsely elevate blood pressure. Getting the child to watch the mercury rise and fall can be helpfully distracting.

In the newborn, especially if sick, doppler ultrasonic methods or oscillometric methods provide the most accurate and reproducible measurements of blood pressure. The flush method is an unreliable measure of blood pressure.

In infancy, the standard auscultatory method can be used with patience and perseverance. By and large toddlers do not like having blood pressure recorded, and there is a dearth of good data in this age group.

From age 5 years blood pressure is easily recorded in children, and some commentators are now suggesting that it be recorded annually — not necessarily to detect abnormality but to establish normality. A range of cuff widths — 7 cm, 9 cm, 11 cm and 13 cm, will be required. We use the simple rule that the largest cuff which fits comfortably around the arm should be applied. The child should be the recipient of any doubt concerning blood pressure recording.

Normal systolic blood pressure

Age (years)	Systolic BP (mm.Hg)	Standard deviation	Upper limit of normal (+2SD)
0.1 (neonate)	60–70	10	90
1–4 (toddler)	90	10	110
6	100	10	120
8	105	10	125
10	110	10	130
12	115	10	135
14	120	10	140

Alternatively, systolic BP = 100 mm. Hg at age 6 years. BP rises by approximately 2.5 mm/year thereafter. (From Report of Task Force on blood pressure control in children. Paediatrics 1977 59: 803.)

Some 'rounding off' of standard deviation and other figures has been done for easier memorability. None of the figures quoted differs significantly from 'Task Force' values.

Normal diastolic blood pressure

Age (years)	Diastolic BP (mmHg)	Standard deviation	Upper limit of normal (+2SD)
2	62	8	78
4	64	8	80
6	66	8	82
8	70	8	86
10	72	8	88
12	74	8	90
14	76	8	92

Or 60 + age in years = approximately mean diastolic. (From Report of Task Force on Blood pressure control in children. Paediatrics 1977 59: 803.)

Some minor 'rounding off' of standard deviation and other figures has been done for easier memorability.

Up to the age of 12 years there are no appreciable differences between boys' and girls' blood pressure.

The heart

Having documented pulse rate, volume, blood pressure, colour, respiratory rate and effort, one may proceed toward the heart. Here the classical skills of inspection, palpation, percussion and auscultation apply. We shall only refer to findings applicable to children.

Inspection

Here one is seeking two major things:
- a precordial bulge and
- visible ventricular impulse.

A precordial bulge will cause the sternum and ribs to bow forwards giving the chest an overblown appearance. The right ventricular impulse may be visible under the xiphisternum. The left ventricular impulse (or apex beat) is frequently visible in thin children, in children with hyperdynamic circulation (due to fever or excitement) and in children with true left ventricular enlargement.

Palpation

Palpation implies localization of the apex beat, a search for right or left ventricular enlargement, and an appreciation of palpable sounds or murmurs. A palpable murmur is referred to as a *thrill*.

Right ventricular enlargement is best sought with one's finger tips placed between 2–3–4th ribs along the left sternal edge. The abnormal palpation in right ventricular hypertrophy is called a tap or a lift. The apex beat is found in the 4th intercostal space along the midclavicular (or nipple) line in infants and toddlers. It may be difficult to localize in plump, healthy infants and toddlers. If you cannot locate the apex beat, think of dextrocardia or a pericardial effusion (both rare phenomena).

In schoolchildren the apex beat is in the 4–5th left intercostal space in the midclavicular line. Left ventricular hypertrophy can result in a diffuse, forceful and displaced apex beat. The feeling is described as a heave.

Palpation of a thrill is always significant. A thrill in the suprasternal notch may suggest coarctation or aortic stenosis. A palpable heart sound usually implies accentuation of that sound (usually pulmonary second sound). Palpation may reveal whether the heart is active or hyperdynamic.

Percussion

We do not find percussion of the heart particularly helpful. However you may be asked to demonstrate cardiac percussion in an examination. The technique is as for an adult.

Auscultation

Auscultation, as stated earlier, should always be left to last, remembering then the old adage — 'sounds first, murmurs second'. In so far as students are concerned the majority of murmurs are systolic until proved otherwise. If you can appreciate diastolic murmurs at the fast heart rates of infancy, you are well tuned into auscultation. We do not propose to reiterate the routine of cardiac auscultation, which is the same at all ages.

When listening:
- try to ensure the child is not crying
- use both diaphragm and bell (preferably paediatric sizes)
- listen in lying and sitting position
- note any variation with respiration.

Sounds first. The first sound is best heard at the apex with the bell and the second at the base with the diaphragm. In infancy, the first sound may be louder than the second. A soft first sound is an early sign of carditis. The first sound may be normally split.

The second sound is normally split in children, this split being physiological and widening on inspiration. A third heart sound may be normal finding in some children.

Murmurs. In so far as students are concerned paediatric murmurs pose two problems:

- hearing them at all
- distinguishing between significant and innocent murmur.

When listening for murmurs try to wipe out all extraneous noise and listen between the first and second sounds *very carefully*, using both diaphragm and bell in all cardiac areas. It is usual to grade murmurs 1–6 in an arbitrary fashion for recording purposes. We propose the following simple system:

Murmur mnemonic:

Grade 1: barely audible; innocent
Grade 2: soft, variable; innocent usually
Grade 3: easy to hear, intermediate, no thrill
Grade 4: loud, audible to anybody, thrill
Grade 5: sounds like a train, very significant, thrill
Grade 6: scarcely requires a stethoscope, thrill.

Murmurs of grades 4–6 are always significant. Grades 1–2 are usually innocent, and grade 3 is intermediate. The length of the murmur is important, pansystolic implying significance, midsystolic suggesting innocence.

Innocent murmurs (also known as physiological, ejection, or flow murmurs) are very common in childhood (being heard in up to 50%) of children. Their distinguishing features are displayed below.

Innocent murmurs are usually:

- midsystolic
- soft in intensity (grade 1–3)
- localized
- poorly conducted
- musical or vibratory in character
- variable with position and respiration
- not associated with other signs of heart disease.

Significant murmurs are usually:

- pansystolic
- conducted all over precordium
- soft to loud (grade 4–6) in intensity

- associated with a thrill
- accompanied by other signs, e.g. ventricular enlargement
- any diastolic.

One innocent murmur which may cause difficulty is the *venous hum*. This is a low-pitched, continuous, rumbling murmur, best heard under the right clavicle. It is usually louder when sitting up, diminishes on lying, and may be abolished by obliterative pressure over the internal jugular vein.

The first hurdle for the student is to distinguish significant murmurs from innocent murmurs. Clearly all murmurs must be properly described — systolic, diastolic, loudness, duration, point of maximal intensity, conduction, etc. Diastolic murmurs are relatively infrequent in children and so require extraordinary auscultatory care if they are to be heard. If the student can determine that the murmur is significant, the next step will be to determine its origin. This will require consideration of colour, pulses, ventricular impulses, heart sounds and the characteristics of the murmur. At undergraduate level, examiners are usually content with elicitation and elucidation of murmurs. If pressed towards a diagnosis, the following points may help.

- cyanosis + murmur: usually Fallot's tetralogy
- cyanosis + murmur + operation: possibly Fallot's tetralogy or transposition of great arteries
- pink + loud systolic murmur: probable ventricular septal defect (the single commonest form of CHD)
- pink + murmur + impalpable femorals: probable coarctation of aorta
- continuous low pitched murmur: possible patent ductus arteriosus.

THE ABDOMEN

In this section we propose to discuss the routine examination of the abdomen, including the genitalia and rectum. We will not refer to palpation or auscultation of the 'acute surgical abdomen'. First a few words on vomiting.

Vomiting

Requires definition. In terms of amount, remember that mothers and nurses tend to overestimate volume of vomitus. What is its frequency and timing? What does it contain — undigested milk, blood, food, bile? Is it forceful or effortless? Try to distinguish projectile vomiting from regurgitant, apparently effortless vomiting. Separate small 'spits' from true vomits. All babies vomit occasionally. Is the vomiting related to feeds? Are feeding volumes appropriate? Is he hungry after he vomits? — the statement 'he's still hungry despite the vomiting' is very characteristic of pyloric stenosis. Does the vomiting bother him? Does the vomiting bother his mother? What has she done about it?

Inspection

The abdomen in toddlers and children is usually protuberant in the upright posture. Even experienced physicians have difficulty distinguishing a normal 'pot-belly' from pathological one. Abdominal protrusion is often related to exaggerated lordosis in the upright position.

Respiration is normally abdominal in type up to school-going age. Small umbilical hernias are a frequent finding. Slight separation (divarication) of the rectus muscles is normal. Distended veins may be noted. Visible loops of bowel are sometimes noted in malnourished infants.

Epigastric hernias are infrequent. By contrast inguinal hernias are common, especially in the male infants. Intra-abdominal masses are occasionally visible. Wilms' tumours can come to medical attention when parents note the swelling on bathing their child.

Abdominal distension is often gaseous. Simple percussion can help to distinguish between solid, cystic and gaseous distension.

Palpation

It is of prime importance to have the infant and child relaxed when trying to palpate the abdomen. This will require patience, skill and distraction techniques. Hands must be warm. Try to avoid making the child cry! You may occasionally have to palpate the abdomen with the infant crawling. Some

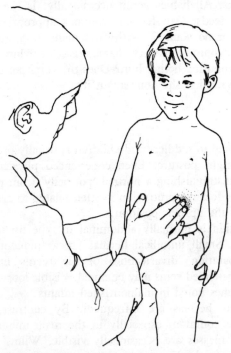

Fig. 5.8 Palpating the abdomen of the toddler standing on a couch.

toddlers will allow you to palpate their abdomens while standing, but object vociferously once you lie them down.

The purpose of abdominal palpation is:
1. To seek the presence of normal abdominal structures.
2. To detect enlargement of abdominal organs.
3. To seek abnormal masses or fluid.

Feeling the spleen

The spleen is to be found in the left upper abdominal quadrant and is normally palpable 1–2 cm below the left costal margin in infancy. It is soft and can be tipped on inspiration.

The enlarged spleen moves on respiration, is dull to percussion, has a notch and one cannot get above it. Don't poke for spleens. Lay you right hand gently on the abdomen and allow the spleen to come to meet it, with your left hand below. Splenic size should be recorded in centimetres below the costal margin. Very large spleens can be missed, if one fails to begin palpation below the umbilicus and work slowly

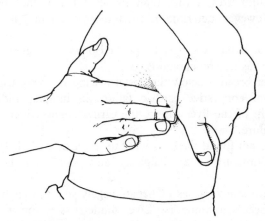

Fig. 5.9 Palpating the spleen.

upwards. The splenic notch is occasionally visible. With chronic enlargement the spleen will usually become firmer. It is rarely tender. The spleen may enlarge medially towards the umbilicus or downwards toward the left iliac fossa. Splenic enlargement tends to be directly downward in infancy.

Palpating the liver

A liver 1–2 cm below the left costal margin is considered normal up to the age of 2–3 years. The liver when enlarged is easily palpable in infants and children. Its edge is soft and it moves down with respiration.

When palpating for the liver *don't poke* as this will provoke tightening of the abdominal muscles. Approach from the RIF with the tips of the fingers or the side of the index finger, lay one's fingers gently on the abdomen and allow the child's respiratory movement to bring the liver to meet your fingers.

Measure liver breadth in centimetres, *not* fingers. It can be useful to percuss out liver dullness and to express total liver size in centimetres, rather than its level below the costal margin. However, determining the upper border may not be easy.

A normal sized liver may be pushed down by a flattened diaphragm, as in bronchoiolitis.

The liver breadth below the costal maring is a very useful indicator of congestive cardiac failure in infants. Indeed enlargement of the liver can be the earliest sign of incipient cardiac failure.

We have not found the *scratch test* to be particularly helpful in determining liver size. Palpation and percussion should suffice.

There are many causes of hepatomegaly in children from storage diseases to tumours. Liver tenderness is sometimes seen in acute hepatitis.

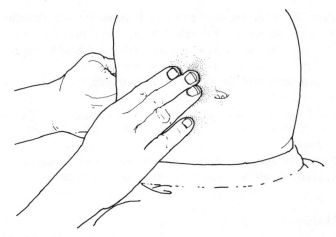

Fig. 5.10 Palpating the liver.

In summary the liver is characterized by the following:
- a palpable edge in the right hypochondrium
- movement with respiration
- dullness to percussion
- inability to get above the swelling.

Palpable nodules and audible bruits over the liver are distinctly unusual in paediatrics. Liver smallness (or atrophy) is almost impossible to clinically designate in children, since inability to palpate a liver is not in itself abnormal.

The kidneys

The kidneys are not easily palpable in infants and children, despite the claims by some authors. Indeed we would say to the inexperienced student — if you can palpate the kidneys they are probably enlarged.

In the hypotonic newborn the kidneys (especially the lower pole) should be palpable and ballotable. Kidneys move on respiration, have a smooth outline, and one can get above them. Kidneys are best palpated bimanually; we have not been impressed by the technique of using the thumbs on anterior approach. The normal fetal lobulation of the newborn kidney is not clinically appreciable.

Enlargement of the kidney in the newborn may be bilateral or unilateral. If unilateral consider congenital meso-nephroma/nephroblastoma (Wilm's), multicystic dysplasia, hydronephrosis, renal vein thrombosis (where the kidney is strikingly firm). If bilateral, renal enlargement may indicate polycystic disease, bilateral obstructive uropathy (secondary to urethral valves), congenital nephrotic syndrome.

Bladder

The bladder can be palpated in the neonate and infant (since it is an abdominal organ) and is easily percussible when full.

Genitalia

Inspection and examination of the genitalia is a routine part of examination of infants, toddlers and school children. More is learnt by inspection than by palpation.

In the male one is looking for normality (or deviation there-from) of the penis, scrotum and testes. Many 'undescended testes' are found on re-examination to represent retractile testes; the over-hasty approach of cold hands has induced a brisk cremasteric reflex. Indeed any self-respecting testis will 'run for cover' if approached threatingly in this fashion. Don't attack the testes!

Is the urethral orifice at the normal position on the tips of the glans? If not is there epispadias (dorsal opening) or hypospadias (ventral opening). Hypospadias may be glandular (common) or penile (rare) or perineal (very rare) (see p. 43).

Male

Enlargement of the *penis* occurs in certain endocrine and neurological conditions. Note that in congenital adrenal hyperplasia the penis is large, but testicular volume is normal. The commonest explanation of a small penis is a normal penis buried in fat. True micropenis (where there may be little palpable other than penile skin and urethra) is rare. Normal penile lengths and circumferences have been published.

Inspection of the *scrotum* should reveal normal rugosity and visible testes. In toddlers and boys testes are best examined in the standing position. The next choice is lying flat on the couch, and the final attempt is made with the child in a squatting position.

1. standing
2. lying
3. squatting

The squatting position helps to abolish the cremasteric reflex and is most valuable in those cases of retractile testes.

A small, flat, underdeveloped scrotum may signify true maldescent. If uncertain about undescended testes always repeat the examination. Undescended testes are a common finding in preterm infants.

Knowledge of normal testicular volume is an attribute not obtained by most practitioners; all that is required is an appreciation of approximate normality. Prader (of Zurich) has produced an orchidometer (or 'testicular rosary') giving a range of testicular volumes.

Awareness of testicular volume may be important, for example, in assessing children with leukaemia (the testes may be a site of relapse), or in following a surgically corrected torsion of the testis (is the testis growing normally?).

Enlargement of the scrotum may be due to an enlarged testis, a hydrocele (transilluminable) or an inguinal hernia. Hydroceles are common in neonates.

Female

The vulva is usually inspected in females. Adhesions of the labial mucosa are not infrequent. Vaginal palpation is *not* usually performed unless there are clear cut clinical indications, such as suspected foreign body, suspected sexual abuse, vaginal discharge, etc.

The clitoris is prominent in preterm infants. A bloody postnatal vaginal discharge ('newborn period') is an occasional normal event. The uterus and ovaries are not normally palpable in infants and children.

Come to terms: Abdomen

atresia	= closed lumen
omphalocele (exomphalos)	= midline hernia containing abdominal contents, sac covers
gastroschisis	= paramedian hernia, no sac
urachus	= embryological connection from bladder to umbilicus

Examining for ascites

Ascites in the newborn may be:
- a transudate, as in hydrops, heart failure
- an exudate, in peritonitis
- biliary (rupture of common bile duct)
- urinary (spontaneous or traumatic rupture of the bladder)
- chylous (rupture of lymphatic duct).

Of the above, only a transudate is in anyway common. Ascites is also seen in chronic liver disease and is a fairly frequent accompaniment of the nephrotic syndrome in childhood.

The ability to demonstrate ascites is frequently sought by examiners, and is therefore an important clinical skill to acquire correctly.

Gross ascites:

- may be obvious on *inspection*
- the abdomen is distended
- the umbilicus is everted
- there are obvious pressure marks on the skin
- the flanks are full
- the skin looks oedematous, and
- the vulva or scrotum are full.

A 'fluid thrill' is an unreliable sign, and can easily be elicited (incorrectly) in very obese children. More reliable by far is the sign of 'shifting dullness'. In looking for dullness one should percuss from resonant (above) to dullness (below). If there is definite dullness in the flank, the child should be rolled onto one side, and a change to resonant percussion note sought — 'shifting dullness'. One must be careful not to percuss over the iliac crest in determining flank dullness. The distribution of ascitic dullness is 'horseshoe-shaped'.

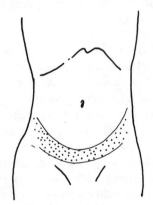

Fig. 5.11 Distribution of ascitic fluid.

Putting your finger in the rectum

Rectal examination need not be routine in children. Always explain to children before you do it. Tell him you hate doing it, but have to. Always use lubrication. Relax the child as best you can. Rectal examination is most often done in acute abdomens, chronic constipation, and rectal bleeding. Use the little finger for little children (neonates and infants) and index finger for older children. Lie the child on his side with legs drawn up. Approach the rectum from the inferior always taking the opportunity to inspect the perianal area prior to inserting one's finger. One occasionally may see threadworms, skin tags or protruding polyps. Haemorrhoids are rare in children. On spreading the buttocks apart, anal fissure may become apparent. Anal fissures (fissure-in-ano) are most often seen at 6 and 12 o'clock and may be accompanied by sentinel tags.

On insertion of one's finger anal tone can be easily assessed. A tight anus resisting one's finger is suggestive of anal stenosis. A loose patulous anus usually indicates a lower spinal lesion such as myelomeningocele or diastematomyelia.

In examining the rectum one is looking primarily for:
- masses (faeces, polyps, teratomas)
- local abdominal tenderness
- blood or other staining on the examining glove.

There are mixed surgical opinions on the value of rectal examination in the clinical situation of 'acute abdomen? appendicitis' in children. We would suggest that it is a useful procedure as one may detect tenderness (in a retrocaecal appendix) and occasionally an appendix mass.

Rectal prolapse and rectal polyps are infrequent findings in paediatrics. While children put foreign bodies in all sorts of orifices, rectal foreign bodies are very unusual. Mothers occasionally bring in roundworms and tapeworms which have been passed per rectum; these should always be kept for proper identification.

Inspection of the underwear and perianal region is important in the child with faecal staining and soiling. Rectal examination may be valuable in distinguishing between constipation with overflow incontinence ('spurious diarrhoea') where the rectum is full of hard faeces, and behavioural soiling where one finds soft faeces in the rectum.

The anus should always be inspected in the newborn to ensure that it is perforate; imperforate anus is easily missed especially in the female who may pass meconium through a vaginal fistula. Hirschprung's disease is among the causes of neonatal intestinal obstruction — the explosive release of flatus is said to be characteristic.

The 'anal wink' or anocutaneous reflex which is contraction of the anus on stroking the perianal region, should be sought in infants with spina bifida.

Other abdominal findings

1. *Faecal masses* can be felt in the central and left lower abdominal quadrants. Sometimes referred to as 'faecal rocks' they are mobile, indentable and non-tender. Remember that immobile children, particularly with severe cerebral palsy, frequently become constipated.

2. *Trichobezoar* (a hair ball) is a rare finding in the stomach of disturbed children.

3. *Tumours*: large tumour masses include nephroblastoma, neurotblastoma, cystic teratoma, hepatoblastoma, mesenteric cysts. These are most often found in infants and toddlers.

4. *Ovaries* are not usually palpable in girls. Enlarged palpable ovaries are associated with ovarian cysts, teratomas and tumours.

5. *Adrenal glands* are never palpable, even though relatively large in the newborn. Enlargement of the adrenal is a feature of tumours usually phaeochromocytoma and neuroblastoma.

EXAMINING THE GLANDS

Children are frequently brought to doctors because of cervical lymph nodes whose apparent persistent enlargement can be a source of concern to parents. Neck glands may be readily visible in thin children. Needless to remark, an unspoken fear of leukaemia may initiate the consultation. Most often these 'swollen glands' are normal, reflect recent infection, and need not cause worry. Small, pea-sized, discrete, non-tender, shotty glands are a normal finding in the cervical and inguinal chains in preschool children. Inguinal glands are occasionally palpable in newborn infants.

Enlarged unilateral axillary glands are often felt after neonatal BCG vaccination. They are usually due to local inflammation/infection at the injection site. Rarely one sees tuberculous axillary lymphadenitis after BCG.

Examination of the lymphoreticular system is an integral part of the examination of the child. One may either systematically go over areas where lymph nodes may be felt, or seek them during examination of individual body systems. We suggest that lymph nodes are best palpated in a methodical, systematic fashion from 'top to toe' — it takes but a short time.

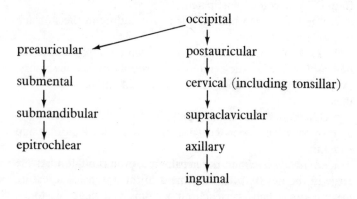

Neck glands should be examined from both behind and in front of the child. Site, size, consistency, tenderness, mobility and attachments of nodes should be carefully recorded. The diameter of single enlarged nodes should be noted. If many lymph glands are enlarged one must always look for splenomegaly and hepatomegaly.

Persistent enlargement of cervical lymph nodes usually reflects acute tonsillitis. While acute tonsillitis subsides rapidly, the draining nodes take much longer to do so. Children with atopic eczema frequently have enlarged regional lymph nodes. Generalized lymph node enlargement should initiate a search for acute infection, inflammation or neoplastic process (see below):

Cervical lymphadenopathy:
- tonsillitis, pharyngitis, sinusitis
- chronic gingivosto matitis
- 'glandular fever' (infectious mononucleosis/cytomegalovirus)
- tuberculosis (uncommon in developed world).

Generalized lymphadenopathy:
- acute exanthemata
- 'glandular fever'
- systemic juvenile chronic arthritis (Still's disease)
- acute lymphatic leukaemia
- drug reaction
- mucocutaneous lymph node syndrome (Kawasaki syndrome).

EAR, NOSE, MOUTH AND THROAT

The ear

The ear is *low-set* when the helix (top of the pinna) meets the cranium at a level below that of a horizortal plane with the corner of palpebral fissure. Pain on pulling the pinna suggests a boil in the external canal. Many mothers suggest that children with otitis media 'pulls their ears' or that the pinna is red in middle ear infections.

Abnormalities of the pinna are seen in many syndromes, from Treacher–Collins to Down's syndrome. It has been said, but not substantiated, that abnormalities of the external ear are associated with kidney abnormalities; the association is a weak one. Cosmetic abnormalities such as protruding ('bat ears') are common. Large ears have been described in the 'fragile X' syndrome.

Examining the ear drums

It must be said that otoscopy is frequently poorly performed by students — they rush at the child, fail to instruct the mother properly, use too small a speculum and sometimes hurt the child.

The mother should gently but firmly hold the child against her chest, one hand over forhead, the other hand around the chest grasping the child's hands. The legs may be held between the mother's thighs if necessary.

In the infant the pinna should be pulled downwards since the canal is directed upwards. In the older child pull the ear up to direct the drum towards the visualizing otoscope. Not infrequently wax will obscure one's view. Should it be removed? Certainly not by the inexpert student.

Always use the largest speculum you expect to fit. We prefer the penhold grip as this allows the otoscope to move readily with any movement of the child. Inspect the canal on the way in.

If the child is fearful of otoscopy, demonstrate it first on the mother. Do not push the otoscope in more than 0.5 cm in infants or 1 cm in older children. One may see otitis externa or a furuncle (exquisitely painful) in the canal. One

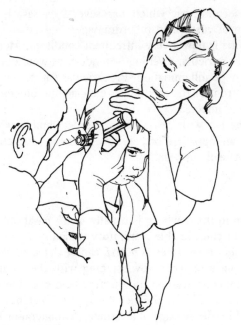

Fig. 5.12 Examining the ear.

occasionally comes across an unexpected foreign body, such as a bead.

The normal appearance of the drum is greyish-white and translucent with a clear light reflex. The most common abnormality to detect is redness, which if accompanied by bulging, implies middle ear infection.

Pinkness or redness of the drum is readily determined. Remember that crying may suffuse the drum and give the false impression of 'inflammation'. We have been impressed by the difficulty in locating perforations when pus is exuding from the canal.

A dull, retracted or full drum with loss of light reflex is indicative of serous otitis media (commonly known as 'glue ear'). This condition, which has several causes, is due to obstruction of eustachian tube drainage.

Mastoiditis is now a very infrequent condition. More likely today a post auricular swelling or tenderness would be caused by lymph node inflammation. Preauricular sinuses or pits can be seen in front of the ear; they are congenital but sometimes may become infected.

Treat the ear with restraint and respect and it will repay you with an appreciation of how redness, retraction and perforation really appear.

The nose

Respiration in the newborn is usually *nasal*; nasal obstruction can result in considerable respiratory difficulty, even apnoea. Air movement through each nostril can be detected by feeling flow with one's fingertip, by listening with the stethoscope, or by noting condensation on a mirror held over the anterior nares. If in doubt, in the newborn, nasal patency can be established by the passage of a catheter. Unilateral or bilateral choanal atresia is a rare finding.

A flat nasal bridge is usually normal. However, it is a notable feature of Down's syndrome.

The nose is a common receptacle for foreign bodies (beads, etc) which may result in unilateral purulent discharge. The nose may be examined using the auriscope — gently. A boggy nasal mucosa may suggest allergy. Nasal polyps sugggest asthma or cystic fibrosis. A chronic, mucopurulent nasal discharge through the winter is a frequent finding in cold climates.

A common complaint concerns the child with persistent nasal discharge ('runny nose'). The discharge may be clear (as in viral or allergic rhinitis) or purulent (suggesting sinusitis or adenoidal obstruction). Bloody nasal discharge (epistaxis) often results from nose picking. Spontaneous epistaxis usually originates from a minor vascular malformation of the nasal mucosa (Little's area). Parents (understandably) exaggerate blood loss in epistaxis.

The mouth

The oral cavity is hostile and often unexplored territory to innocent practitioners, paediatric and general alike. Mouths that won't open, jaws clamped on a prising spatula, teeth ready to snap on probing fingers, a fleeting glimpse at tonsils and quivering uvula. Infants and small children do not like to have their mouths and throats examined. Hence this examination should be left until just about last. Some will open as wide as a yawning alligator on the promise that a spatula

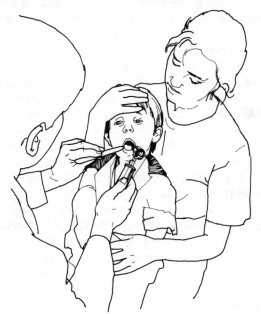

Fig. 5.13 Examining the mouth and throat.

will not be used. Others have to be coaxed into co-operation. Sometimes pressing a finger into each cheek will force open the mouth. When necessary the child could be appropriately restrained (Fig. 5.13).

Proper inspection of the tonsils requires a good light source, a well opened mouth and a speedy observer.

The *tonsils* can be surprisingly difficult to visualize in neonates and infants as the tongue seems always to ride up. It is remarkably and embarrassingly easy to miss a cleft of the soft palate in the newborn. One occasionally comes across a bifid uvula of no great consequence.

One has a few fleeting moments to observe redness, exudate, or secretions in the oropharynx. The classical streptococcal tonsillitis produces a unilateral or bilateral follicular exudate. A creamy, confluent exudate is typical of infectious mononeucleosis; other noteworthy features of this illness are palatal petechiae and a swollen uvula. Some texts state that infectious mononucleosis does not occur in young children; this has not been our experience. Diphtheria, though now rare, must not be forgotten. It causes a severe lymphadenitis, 'bull neck', a greyish membrane and notable toxicity. It needs to be stated that gonococcal tonsillitis may have to be considered in atypical or unresponsive infections in adolescents.

While examining the tonsils the student should also look at the oropharynx for evidence of pharyngitis, exudate or a postnasal drip. Postnasal drip may be elicited by asking the child to say 'aah' at length.

Tonsillar size is not important unless extreme. By extremely large tonsils we mean tonsils that meet in the midline (sometimes referred to as 'kissing tonsils'). Repeatedly infected tonsils may have a pitted appearance.

The tongue

A large protruding tongue is a feature of congenital hypothyroidism. Macroglossia may also be caused by a local lymphatic or vascular anomaly. The tongue may appear inappropriately large for a small mouth as in Down's syndrome.

A white coated tongue is usually attributable to a recent milk feed. Monilial infection (thrush) is manifest by a patchy white exudate which cannot easily be removed by a spatula. Herpetic stomatitis affects the tongue, mucosa and buccal border. It is vascular, friable, bleeds to touch, and is associated with marked drooling.

Come to terms: oral cavity

ranula	= cyst on anterior floor of mouth
quinsy	= peritonsillar abscess
glossoptosis	= backward displacement of tongue
micrognathia	= small chin

Buccal mucosa

Thrush appears as serpiginous white patches on the mucosa. Koplik's spots are like a grain of salt with a red rim; they are found in the buccal gutter during measles prodrome. Inflammation of the parotid duct usually implies acute viral parotitis (mumps). Recurrent suppurative parotitis (with or without stone) is a rarity in childhood.

The teeth

Dentists have a modicum of medicine. Doctors have a minimal knowledge of dentisty which is virtually absent from most medical curricula. Particularly in early childhood, the doctor has a unique opportunity to practice some preventive dentistry. Even a brief look into the child's oral cavity and a scan of teeth and gums is a useful exercise. Below are some spin-offs of dental examination:

1. Dental caries is prevalent still, especially in the less well off segments of society. Caries of the upper incisors is sometimes called 'nursing bottle caries'.

2. Early detection of maleruption, malocclusion, and malalignment.

3. Dental staining may be of diagnostic significance. Dental enamel hypoplasia has been described as a sequel of neonatal hypocalcaemia. Brown or yellow staining (which fluoresces under Wood's light) is a side effect of tetracycline consumption in pregnancy and early childhood. Black staining of the teeth sometimes follows iron ingestion.

4. Flattened teeth seen in handicapped children who grind their teeth (bruxism).

5. Absence of teeth is a feature of ectodermal dysplasia.

6. Gingivitis is frequently associated with caries. Gingival hypertrophy, with or without gingivitis, occurs in children consuming phenytoin long term.

SKIN, HAIR AND NAILS

In this section we plan to mention some normal skin variations, some clinical clues to be found in skin, hair and nails, and to propose that the secret of success in skin conditions lies in inspection, palpation and description. We shall not refer to acute infectious exanthemata.

Skin

Skin colour. Discussion of racial variations in skin colour is beyond our remit. Students will be aware of increasing cross racial relationships allowing for all sorts of pigmentary variations.

Mongolian blue spots are black or navy areas over sacrum,

buttocks and sometimes shins of infants from Middle Eastern, African and Asian parents. Pigmentation of the scrotum may be an associated finding.

Absence of skin pigmentation occurs in albinism, which is easily missed at birth as the pink lens may not be noted and skin pigment is light in most infants. Skin pigmentation increases through infancy.

Freckles (multiple small pigmented spots) are fairly common, especially in fair-skinned people.

Café-au-lait spots are pigmented patches more than 1.5 cm in diameter. When greater than six in number they may suggest neurofibromatotis; axillary freckles are characteristic of this condition.

Small *bruises* on the forehead are a normal finding in toddlers, who have recently acquired the skill of walking. Similar small bruises (as many as ten) are a frequent finding on the knees and shins of preschool and schoolchildren. The characteristic sites and appearance of bruises suggestive of nonaccidental injury are described elsewhere (see Appendix 11.11).

Yellow discolouration of the skin — *carotenaemia* — has been described in infants and children consuming excessive amounts of carrots and mandarin oranges.

Vitiligo is an area of depigmented skin, and may be seen in tuberous sclerosis.

Come to terms: hair/skin

hirsutism	= excessiveness hairiness; synonym hypertrichosis
hyperhydrosis	= excessive sweatiness
lentigines	= brownish pigmented spots on skin
vitiligo	= depigmented patches

Sclerema is an erythematous thickening and hardening of the skin associated with hypothermia or vascular stasis. Local sclerema is usually confined to hands and feet. Generalized sclerema indicates a serious systemic disorder.

Generalized *oedema* of the skin is a normal finding in preterm infants. Hydropic conditions of the newborn are accompanied by generalized pitting oedema. Dependent oedema is unusual in the newborn but may occur in the propped infant in congestive cardiac failure.

Lymphpoedema (non-pitting) is classically found in the lower limbs in Milroy's syndrome (congenital lymphoedema) and in the X0 neonate (Turner's syndrome).

Hair

Hair colour, thickness and distribution are racial attributes. Soft downy hair (lanugo) is found in preterm infants. Bushy head hair at birth is a normal variant, but may suggest congenital hypothyroidism. Bushy eyebrows are a feature of mucopolysacharroidoses and of De Langes syndrome. Long eyelashes are a normal (sought after) attribute in girls; they also occur in children with chronic debilitating disorders.

Prominent dark hair on forearms, nape of neck, and back is a normal variant. White flecks in the scalp hair are a feature of de Waardenburg's syndrome. Kinky hair is described in the rare Menkes' syndrome. Lank 'lifeless' hair is sometimes noticed in coeliac disease.

Absent or short occipital hair may be a feature of infants who are either delayed or deprived; it reflects too much time spent in the supine position. Children with Down's syndrome typically have straight hair. Total absence of hair is seen in ectodermal dysplasia (a rare condition), and as a side effect of cytotoxic drugs.

Local absence of hair in a child may reflect either alopecia or trichillomania (hair pulling). In alopecia the area may be totally bald; in trichillomania short hair roots are usually present.

Nits (pediculosis capitis) are a common finding nowadays. They are adherent to hair shafts, difficult to displace and need to be distinguished from dandruff. A paediatric predecessor of ours used to refer to head lice as 'mechanized dandruff'.

Excessive hair (hypertrichosis, hirsutism) may be a side-effect of several drugs including phenytoin, diazoxide, minoxidil and cyclosporin A.

Nails

Nails are often long in the post-term (postmature) newborn infant. Absence of nails is a feature of ectodermal dysplasia. Peripheral cyanosis of nail beds (acrocyanosis) is a normal newborn variant.

Spoon-shaped nails (koilonychia) are occasionally a normal variant; they may be associated with anaemia. White lines across the nails (leuconychia) can be seen with chronic hypoalbuminaemic states, such as nephrotic syndrome and liver disorders. Small white spots on the nails do not indicate calcium deficiency.

Pitting of the nails is described in fungal diseases and in psoriasis. Nail biting is a frequent finding in children, stressed and unstressed.

The secret of success in skins

The secret of success in dermatology is to describe what you see. Stand back, look carefully at the rash and apply descriptive terms to its colour, appearance, distribution, feel, etc. Too many students take one look, and jump at a diagnosis like a salmon at flies. It is better by far to use one's power of description and palpation.

Today's students can be inhibited by a lack of or even a

smattering of Latin or Greek, which certainly helps in understanding skins. The student who knows some Latin would not call the uniform circular lesions of psoriasis 'erythema multiforme'. Included below is a glossary of some classical terms in an effort to overcome confusion.

Glossary of dermatological terminology

erythema	= redness
erythema multiforme	= redness of many shapes
erythema marginatum	= red raised margin
erythema annulare	= red, circular
atopic eczema	= literally means 'out of place boiling over', 'atopy' from 'topos' (Greek for place); eczema = to boil over
centrifugal	= fleeing from the centre
centripetal	= seeking the centre
morbilliform	=. measles-like
varicelliform	= chicken pox-like
ichthyosis	= dry, scaling skin. From ichthus (Greek for fish)

Could we suggest that once you have seen the following rashes that you immediately and carefully describe them:

- psoriasis
- tinea corporis (ringworm)
- erythema nodosum
- anaphylactoid purpura
- molluscum contagiosum.

Describe a rash as though you were attempting to describe it to a blind person — site, size, colour, shape, distribution, feel. Is it a macule, papule or vesicle. Is it itchy? Is it wet or dry? Is it centrifugal or centripetal? Is it raised or flat? What does it feel like?

macule	= flat lesion

papule   = raised lesion
vesicle   = fluid filled lesion
bulla   = a large vesicle
pustule   = vesicle containing pus

Eczema (atopic dermatitis) is the commonest chronic rash in childhood. Eczema is a good example of applying description in order to come to a conclusion. The skin in eczema may be:

- erythematous (red)
- dry
- papular (palpably raised)
- scaling (ichthyotic)
- excoriated (scratched)
- thickened (lichenified)
- weeping (?infected).

In so far as children are concerned, *four irritations of eczema* are:

- itching
- ichthyosis
- infection
- image (of self).

Palpation of the rash is most important and frequently not performed. Few rashes in paediatrics are painful. Measurement of lesions and clinical photography are very useful for recording purposes.

It is important to remember that skin, teeth, hair and nails are all ectodermal structures and should be seen as a continuum particularly when dealing with congenital abnormalities of some part of the system as in ectodermal dysplasia. The state of the hair and skin, in particular, can contribute to a clinical assessment of a child's state of nutrition.

Chilblains (perniosis) are sometimes seen in children living in cold houses in cold climates. They are noted on the fingers, toes and occasionally the ears; they are inflammatory blisters, which may ulcerate.

Intertrigo may be observed in overweight infants and children. This is a wet, red, eruption in furrows between opposed skin surfaces of the groin, axilla and sometimes neck.

In summary examination of any rash must include:
- inspection
- palpation
- good description.

Come to terms: derm

dermatoglyphics	= study of fingerprint and hand crease patterns
dermatographia	= skin writing. White line with red margins following scratching of skin
dermoid	= teratoma of skin structures
dermatophagoides pyterrinissinus	= house dust mite

NEUROLOGICAL EXAMINATION

We do not propose to exhaustively deal with the neurological system, but rather to present some points about the neurological system and its examination that are *different* in infants, toddlers and preschool children. Neurological examination at these ages cannot always be performed in an organized fashion.

By contrast a 'classical' full neurological examination can be carried out on a co-operative schoolchild. It's tricks and techniques are fully described in your basic text on clinical methods so we will not elaborate further. The neurological examination of the newborn is described in Chapter 4. Intrinsic to an understanding of the infant's neurological system is that maturation of the CNS is manifest by a loss of primitive reflexes with a corresponding gain in positive skills. Developmental examination, including speech, hearing, gross and fine movement is presented in Chapter 8.

The neurological approach combines:

1. Careful history of birth, perinatal events, developmental sequence, maternal worries, etc.

2. Observation of the infant's activity, symmetry and of the toddler's movement, play and socialization.

3. Expedient examination of tone, power, coordination, reflexes, sensation. Sensation can be especially difficult to ascertain in infancy.

History

One will need to enquire about movement in utero. While maternal instincts as to normal intrauterine movement may be fallible, in retrospect they may be alerting. Reduced fetal movement may be significant.

Perinatal events are important. Low Apgar scores (< 5) at 1 and 5 minutes, while not in themselves prognostically valuable, may contribute to concern.

How did the baby suck? And move? Did he pass his neonatal neurological examination?

Tell me about his development. Was a normal pattern followed? When did he first smile with meaning? When did he sit unsupported, etc. The modern mother may well have filled these developmental milestones in her baby's book or diary. If so, ask to look at it.

If a mother presents her infant with a possible developmental or neurological problem remember our primary premises:

- she's usually right
- her worries often commenced well before attending doctors
- her instincts are sharper than your observations.

Alerting statements made by mothers include the following:

'He was an unusually good baby' (this may mean he cried or moved very little, but merely slept and fed).

'He was always different from the others'.

'He was okay till 9 months of age then he seemed to stop'.

'He seems to have gone backwards'.

Infant with perinatal insults tend to be abnormal in their behaviour from the beginning. Babies with neurodegenerative disorders, for example, may develop normally for a period and then stop, or indeed, regress.

Neurologists, above all specialists, are obsessive in their demand for a good history. When did the problem begin? What was the child like before that? What exactly happened? What has been the sequence of events since then? Giving a history of a convulsion to a neurologist as an intern is akin to being cross-examined in court by a querulous senior counsel. So learn the art before you qualify. Be confident, be complete and choose your words carefully. In other words, take a good history, or risk being 'hammered'.

Examination techniques

We plan merely to highlight some skills and certain signs particular to paediatrics. For detailed description of neurological examination refer to your text of clinical signs.

Tendon reflexes

The fingertip is sometimes used to elicit knee jerks in neonates; this is acceptable practice. After the newborn period we recommend the use of a small reflex hammer. When striking a tendon with the hammer be a swinger not a stabber — in other words allow the hammer to have a free flowing stroke. The knee jerk is best tapped with the hammer held in a pengrip and parallel to the leg.

Deep tendon reflexes may be arbitrarily graded for record purposes as follows:

0 = absent
1+ = weak response
2+ = normal response
3+ = exaggerated response
4+ = very brisk response.

Exaggerated responses are characteristic of upper motor neurone (pyramidal) lesions, reduced reflexes occur with muscle weakness, and absent reflexes suggest a peripheral neuropathy (lower motor neurone).

Fundoscopy

In infants and toddlers, fundoscopy requires the patience of Job and a fair amount of skill. Fundoscopy can at times be akin to seeking a passenger in a train rushing by. Do your best. Don't be depressed if you fail — we all do (see p. 139 for more detailed discussion).

Neonate

We will only briefly mention the newborn, whose neurological examination is detailed in Chapter 4, Newborn.

Observe the posture adopted by newborn babies and infants. Observe limb movements and in particular whether symmetrical or not. Note the normal flexed position of the well infant. See the 'frog position' of the floppy infant. Look for neck extension in infants with 'cerebral irritation' or with severe meningism. Look for spontaneous movement and for abnormal movements.

Normal newborn findings

- Tremulousness
- Mass responses

- Extensor plantar response
- Unsustained ankle clonus

Babinski response may be upgoing (extensor) to the age of 8 months.

Infant

How does the infant handle? This is an important observation. Does he resent handling (as, for example, infants with meningism)? Is he floppy? — does he tend to slip through your hands in upright suspension? Is he stiff? — does he tend to move 'in one piece'? Is muscle tone decreased?

Cranial nerve examination

Full cranial nerve examination can be difficult in infants and toddlers. However simple tests can achieve a lot as detailed below.

First cranial nerve (olfactory) — almost impossible in preschool children. Second, third, fourth and sixth cranial nerves — see under Eyes.

Fifth cranial nerve — facial sensation requires considerable expertise to examine in toddlers. However, cardinal reflex requires trigeminal nerve function. Corneal reflex likewise.

Activity	Cranial nerves used
Rooting	5
Crying	7
Smiling	7
Sucking	5,7,9
Swallowing	9,10,11
Gag reflex	9
Tongue movement	12

Disappearance of primitive reflexes with appearance of positive skills is part of the developmental sequence. Persistence of primitive reflexes is neurologically sinister.

Primitive reflexes: appearance and disappearance

Placing	Newborn	1 year
Stepping	Newborn	2 months
Moro	Birth	3–5 months
Palmar grasp	Birth	2 months
Plantar grasp	Birth	8–10 months
Asymmetric tonic neck	Newborn	1–6 months

Feeling the fontanelle

If the eye is the window of the soul, the fontanelle is a window on the infant's brain.

The tension of the anterior fontanelle is an important sign in deciding whether or not an infant has raised intracranial pressure and in determining the presence and degree of dehydration. The fontanelle must preferably be palpated (gently!) when the infant is quiet or sitting upright. Fullness and elevation of the fontanelle over the surrounding skull is evidence of increased intracranial pressure. The usual causes of this will be meningitis or hydrocephalus. No comment should be made if the infant is crying.

A systolic bruit is frequently audible over the anterior fontanelle in the presence of meningitis. This usually disappears in 2–3 days.

Delayed closure (beyond 18 months) of the anterior fontanelle is associated with:

- normal variation
- hydrocephalus
- Down's syndrome
- hypothyroidism

- bone disorders
- some syndromes
- arteriovenous malformation.

A rapidly enlarging head may be a cause of concern. Serial measurements of head circumference are important. If a large head is accompanied by a full fontanelle and spread sutures, raised intracranial pressure is the likely cause. Some causes of *large head* are:

- hydrocephalus
- space occupying lesion
- storage diseases
- bone disorders
- familial macrocephaly
- Sotos' syndrome.

Head growth is a reflection of brain growth. However except at the extremes head size is not related to intelligence. Small heads (*below third centile*) are called microcephaly. Some causes of microcephaly include:

- perinatal hypoxia
- intrauterine infection
- chromosomal disorders
- familial
- dysmorphic syndrome
- severe metabolic disorder

Enlarging heads can be sometimes halted; poorly growing heads, unfortunately usually cannot be helped.

Eliciting neck stiffness

Meningism or neck stiffness is a very important sign to elicit correctly. The student needs to be gentle, always to look for passive resistance to flexion before active resistance, and to be aware of voluntary resistance exhibited by that 'enfant terrible', the fretful toddler. It is important to state at the outset that neck stiffness, unless severe and obvious, is an unreliable sign in the neonate and infant.

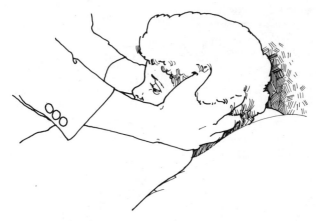

Fig. 5.14 Examining for neck stiffness.

First, observe the infant's position of comfort. The well relaxed child sleeps in a position of cuddled flexion. The ill infant may extend. The infant with severe meningeal irritation may adopt the position of *opisthotonus* or hyperextension of the neck and trunk.

Ask the toddler to follow a light. Ask the child to flex his chin onto his chest. Ask him to kiss his knee. In the sitting position ask him to look at the roof. If he can do all of these readily, neck stiffness is likely to be absent, or if present, minimal.

Then, while supporting his occiput, gently flex his neck feeling for resistance to movement. In severe meningism the child will lift up 'like a board'. Lesser degrees of meningism may cause him to wince or cry on flexion. Always note carefully the facial expression when looking for meningism.

Kernig's sign (resistance to straight leg raising)

This can be elicited in children and has the same significance as in adults. Kernig's sign is, however, unreliable under the

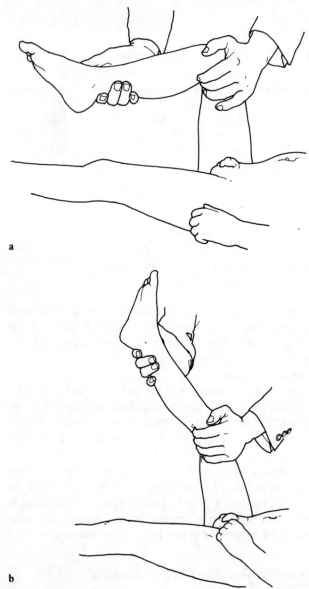

a

b

Fig. 5.15 Kernig's sign.

age of 3 years. Kernig's sign is performed by flexing the hip and knee to a right angle and then slowly extending the leg. A positive sign exists when there is pain and limitation of movement. While doing this maneouvre it is useful to feel for tightness of the hamstring. The child may additionally demonstrate Brudzinski's sign by reciprocally flexing the contralateral knee in order to take the stretch off his lower spine.

Meningism

Genuine meningism is likely to be associated with a shrill, high pitched cry. The infant may be drowsy and irritable, may refuse feeds, and may wish to be left alone. Meningism does not always imply meningitis. It must be recognized that meningism may be associated with upper respiratory and other infections.

Some causes of meningism

- meningitis, encephalitis
- acute otitis media
- severe tonsillitis
- cervical lymphadenitis
- pneumonia
- retropharyngeal abscess

Toddler

In mobile children more is learned by the amateur through informal observation than by formal examination. Observe:

walking	transferring
running	jumping
climbing	scribbling
kicking	smacking (you!)

Clearly, skills achieved in all of these areas will be related to chronological and developmental age. The speed and dexterity with which the above are performed can be very informative. Be prepared to get onto the floor and observe *play*. Play is the all-consuming interest of toddlers and preschool children. You can note constructiveness, concentration, conversation (children often speak to themselves when playing), coordination, and curiosity. A period in the ward playroom will be well repayed. Beneath the apparent chaos, a lot of important business is being carried on. The combination of a good maternal history and a few Lego bricks can help you construct a neurological template. Observe:

- alertness ⎤
- activity ⎬ at all ages
- adaptation ⎦

Note the toddler's *gait*, hand or foot preference (if determined) and in particular look for symmetry of movement. Children with a hemiplegia tend not to want to use the hand on the affected side. Hemiplegia may delay the onset of walking; he drags the leg or limps. All gaits are unsteady for a while after acquisition of walking. Persisting unsteadiness, frequent falls and dropping of objects may suggest ataxia. Observation of play is imperative in determining coordination.

It is worth observing the gait of any child with a suspected neurological disorder. Children usually acquire the skill of independent walking between 10–18 months. The initial gait is unsteady and broad based; confidence and coordination are rapidly gained. Failure to walk independently by 18 months warrants an explanation (familial, obesity, bottom-shuffler?) and an examination to establish normality or determine the cause.

Certain characteristic gaits are worth noting and if possible videorecording:

1. Gait of muscular dystrophy — is of a waddling nature, the hips being thrown from side to side.

2. Ataxic gait — usually wide based, unsteady and poorly coordinated.

3. Hemiplegic gait — tendency to drag and to circumduct the leg with extended foot, which scrapes the ground.

4. Lower limb weakness results in the foot being dragged and a slapping gait.

5. Toe walking gait is not in itself abnormal, and has been noted in infants born prematurely.

6. Possible causes of a limping gait are mentioned on p. 134. Remember that a late or missed congenital dislocation of the hip may not be apparent until the child walks.

Schoolchild (5+ years)

The co-operative schoolchild will usually allow you to carry our a complete formal neurological examination as appropriate. This is described in your text on clinical methods so we will not duplicate. One will always have to make allowance for the child's confidence, co-operation, and comprehension of what is required of him. The examiner will need to be patient, expedient and to be prepared to try again. Testing of children's sensation is not often required but when performed needs clear explanation to the child of the answers being sought (children are very obliging creatures and may give false answers for fear of disappointing you!).

In the schoolchild the following tests of co-ordination are the best:
- one leg stance
- hopping
- straight line walking.

In addition you may wish to observe the child writing, kicking a ball, tying his shoelace, clapping, catching a ball, kicking, buttoning his shirt. By the age of 5 years hand domination is determined — most children are predominantly right-handed, right-footed and right-eyed.

The neurological examination is not complete without a clinical comment on:

- vision
- hearing
- speech
- intelligence.

Come to terms: odd movements

chorea	= coarse, involuntary, purposeless movements
athetosis	= slow, writhing, incoordinate movements
tic	= repeated bizarre movements; habit spasms
tremor	= constant small movement

Determination of tone

Tone implies resistance to passive movement and its assessment is related to age. In the newborn and infant, tone is best assessed by neck traction, by ventral and upright suspension, and passive movement of limb joints. Tone may be normal, reduced (hypotonic or floppy), or increased (hypertonic, spastic). The infant (post neonatal) who 'slips' through your hands in upright suspension is hypotonic. Hypotonia may be caused by muscle weakness or wasting (as in malnutrition, myopathies, cerebellar lesions, and neuropathies). Wrists and ankle joints may be unduly floppy and muscles may feel flabby. Shaking of wrists and ankle joints is a useful index of tone in infants.

The characteristics of spasticity are increased tone of the muscles and exaggerated deep tendon reflexes. One has to work harder to flex and extend the joints involved. Rigidity may be of the 'lead-pipe' variety (the same throughout the range of movement), clasp-knife (stiff initially, but gives), or 'cogwheel type' (jerky throughout).

A selection of CNS signs

1. *Cracked pot note* is the hollow, cracking note one obtains on percussing the skull in the presence of raised intracranial pressure and closed fontanelles. The examiner's ear is applied directly to the head and the skull percussed with one finger. In older children with space occupying lesions and spread sutures a 'hollow note' may be elicited. The sound is quite different from the solid note of the sound skull. The sideroom technique of skull transillumination has been rendered superfluous by the advent of cranial ultrasound.

2. *Setting sun sign* is when the sclera is visible above the iris. It is seen in hydrocephalus with raised intracranial pressure. It is also seen in normal 'pop-eyed' infants.

3. *Head tilt* is an interesting and important sign. It may be evidence of torticollis and is seen in children with strabismus and ptosis. Rarely it has been described as an early sign of an occipital tumour.

4. *Doll's eye reflex* is where the eyes move in the opposite direction to that of the head.

Cerebral palsy

Definition: a disorder of movement and posture presenting in infancy and characterized by one or a combination of hypotonia, spasticity, ataxia, involuntary movements.

The common types of cerebral palsy are:
- hemiplegia ⎫
- quadriplegia ⎬ spastic
- diplegia ⎭
- ataxia
- dyskinesis — choreoathetosis, dystonia.

Hemiplegia

The upper limb is more involved than the lower limb. There

is marked thumb adduction, fisting and increased pronator tone. Contractures may occur and limb growth may be retarded.

Quadriplegia

In this situation all four limbs are involved, particularly the upper. The predominant sign is hypertonia, demonstrable at the wrists and elbows, and also in the ankles, knees and hips.

Diplegia

The lower limbs are more severly involved with a symmetrical distribution. Clinical presentation coincides with development of extension in the lower trunk and hips. Typically the infant drags himself around the floor with flexed arms and extended legs. Extensor spasticity at the hips and knees results in the classical signs of extension and scissoring of lower limbs.

Orthopaedic deformities may result from the altered tone, including:

- kyphosis of the thoracic spine
- lordosis of the lumbar spine
- dislocation of the hips
- equinovarus or valgus feet.

Ataxia

- diplegia (as described above)
- cerebellar involvement
- initial hypotonia
- intention tremor
- stamping gait.

Dyskinesis

This implies irregular and involuntary movements of some or all groups of muscles. These movements may be continuous or be present only when the limb is deliberately moved. The signs of dyskinesis include hypotonia, slow and purposeless movements, involvement of distal parts of limbs, and accentuated voluntary movements.

Disabilities associated with cerebral palsy

- mental handicap (IQ < 70) in 75%
- visual — squint, refractive errors
- hearing — partial deafness
- speech — disorders of sensation, perception and language development
- epilepsy
- emotional problems.

The purpose of physical and neurological examination is to determine:

- the type of cerebral palsy
- the severity and distribution of the problem
- the nature and extent of associated mental and physical handicap.

MUSCULO-SKELETAL SYSTEM

In this section we have arbitrarily lumped together the limbs, muscles, bones and joints, with a few words on congenital malformations. A lot of interesting paediatric case material is to be found on the orthopaedic ward. We propose to highlight a few points in a chronological fashion — newborn, toddler and school child.

A thorough examination is from head to toe. Most students are thorough in their systematic questioning and systems examination. Nonetheless the untrained eye can easily miss little things, which may be relevant — polydactyly, for example, or 2–3rd toe partial syndactyly (a common finding), or 5th finger clinodactyly. We have seen schoolchildren with the Poland syndrome (absence of the pectoralis major muscle and/or nipple) whose parents have failed to notice this apparently obvious deformity. Scoliosis is easily missed at any age unless one specifically looks for it.

Observe the infant or child in his preferred position. If mobile, watch how he moves around. Does he creep, crawl, bottom-shuffle? Observe the gait. Can he run? Note co-ordination, dexterity and symmetry of movement. Can he hop on one foot (a good test of co-ordination as well as muscular strength)? Can he jump? How does he get up from the sitting position?

Has he a limp, waddle or other abnormal gait. Are the limbs symmetrical and of equal length? Parents will frequently seek medical advice on normal postural variations — intoeing (due to metatarsus adductus), bow-leggedness (genu varum) and lumbar lordosis (producing a protuberant abdomen).

Types of abnormality

- malformation = structural defect of an organ or area
- deformation = abnormal form or position of a part due to compression
- disruption = breakdown of otherwise normal developmental process.

Come to terms: orthopaedics

talipes equinovarus	= club foot
genu varum	= bow-legged
genu valgum	= knock-kneed
genu recurvatum	= knees bent backwards
gibbus	= sharply angled kyphosis

Some simple rules when dealing with the painful, limping orthopaedic or arthritic child are listed below.

Orthopaedic rules . . . . OK?
- above all, don't hurt the child
- active movements always before passive
- never force a joint — especially a suspected congenital dislocation of hip
- if in doubt, don't!

The newborn

At this age one's major interest is in detection of congenital abnormality. Are there 10 fingers and 10 toes? Any webs? Are the limbs symmetrical? Any positional deformities? Mild positional deformities of the feet, for example, varus (inturning) or valgus (out-turning) are common. Gentle manipulation will restore the foot to its correct position.

Fixed deformities such as clubfoot (talipes equinovarus) are frequently associated with spina bifida, and will not correct on manipulation.

Congenital dislocation of the hip (see newborn examination, Chapter 4)

The correct technique of the hip examination is important to acquire — the 'Baby-Hippy' may help in this respect. It is vital to remember that if congenital dislocation of the hip is not detected in the newborn period, it may not be evident until walking is attempted at which stage curative correction is difficult. Hip examination is rewarding in the first week, less so at 6 weeks, and unrewarding at 6 months. Whenever you see a young adult female with an evident 'hip-dip' gait you ought to say to yourself? congenital dislocation and resolve to examine babies' hips properly.

Come to terms: fingers/toes

syndactyly	= fusion of digits
clinodactyly	= incurved digit
camptodactyly	= flexed digit
polydactyly	= extra digits
arachnodactyly	= long thin digits

Limb deformities

Limb reduction defects (of the type seen following thalidomide ingestion in pregnancy) are rare and will not be considered in detail. Proper measurement of limb length will be valuable in suspected asymmetry. Precise measurement of the lower limb is from the anterior ischial spine to the lower aspect of the medial malleolus. Hemihypertrophy has important associations with, for example, aniridia (absence of the iris) and nephroblastoma.

Come to terms: limb deformities

amelia	= absence of limb
hemielia	= absence of distal half of limb
phocomelia	= hand or foot attached directly to trunk
arthrogryposis	= curved joints
osteogenesis imperfecta (fragilitas ossium)	= brittle bone disease

Neural tube defects are sufficiently common, particularly in Celtic races, to warrant mention. The defects are usually obvious on inspection, and the associated disabilities and deformities will depend on the site and size of the lesion. The length and width of the lesion should be measured. The different types of neural tube defects are encephalocele, myelomeningocele, meningocele, and spina bifida occulta or dysraphism. In the minor and lower spinal types of spina bifida the clinical signs may be subtle — hairy tuft overlying the spine, 'lipomatous' lump or mild lower limb wasting or weakness. There is a strong association between neural tube defect and hydrocephalus.

Come to terms: neural tube defect

spina bifida	= failure of fusion of cerebral arches (synonym = rachischisis)
meningocele	= open vertebral arches with overlying sac containing CSF
myelomeningocele	= unfused vertebral arches with exposed neural tissue
hydrancephaly	= almost complete absence of cerebral hemispheres
anencephaly	= congenital absence of cranial vault
encephalocele	= herniation of brain through congenital skull defect

The neck

An apparent short neck is common in the newborn. Normal neck movement can be demonstrated by turning the baby's head to 90° on each side.

A fibrous nodule midway along the sternomastoid muscle (sternomastoid 'tumour') is an occasional finding in the neonate. It usually resolves spontaneously.

The thyroid gland is usually neither visible nor palpable in the newborn. An obvious goitre suggests some form of hypothyroidism (secondary to a thyroid enzyme deficiency) or transient hyperthyroidism.

Thyroglossal cysts are rare midline lesions which change position with tongue movement.

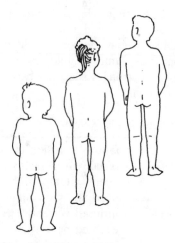

Fig. 5.16 Normal lower limb variations.

Toddler and preschool child

The normal toddler frequently has a mildly bow-legged gait. This may convert to a knock-kneed posture in the preschool age. Neither should cause concern unless extreme. Most toddlers have flat feet. Intoeing is a frequent finding due usually to metatarsus varus or to tibial torsion.

Limp

Limp a frequent clinical problem in small children and will require careful examination of spine, hip, knee and foot.

The approach to the limping child will be based on (a) history, (b) age and (c) clinical examination. The chronology of hip disorders in children has been well described. Inspection of the child's position, gait and lower limb will be imperative. Examination of hip, knee and ankle joint for range of movement will follow. A careful search for local heat or tenderness, for embedded foreign body, and for rash or lumps will be necessary. Among the multiple causes of acute limp in a child one could include the following:

- irritable hip   Perthes' disease
- transient synovitis   slipped femoral epiphysis
- pyogenic arthritis
- osteomyelitis   anaphylactoid purpura
- discitis   lymphatic leukaemia
- osteochondritis   coagulation disorder
- Puncture wound, verruca, foreign body in foot
- Spiral fracture of tibia or fibula
- rheumatoid arthritis
- bone tumour
- trauma
- inguinal hernia
- testicular tarsion.

Muscle strength

This can be difficult to determine in preschool children. Wasted muscles feel flabby and the muscle power may be appropriately reduced. The muscles may look large, but feel rubbery, in Duchenne dystrophy.

Most of us require the assistance of a neurologist or physiotherapist in grading the strength of groups of muscles in preschool children.

Gower's sign

Gower's sign (where the child 'climbs up' his legs from the reclining position) is a classical sign of muscular dystrophy but is seen in other forms of muscle weakness.

Muscle tenderness

This is indicative of myositis. Acute viral myositis with

refusal to walk, tenderness of the calf muscles, and little constitutional upset is a recognized clinical entity. It is seen usually in children aged 5–10 years.

Schoolchild

In this section we propose to selectively mention (a) joint examination (b) arthritis and (c) examination for scoliosis.

The systematic examination of muscles, joints and bones in the schoolchild is as for an adult. Limb or joint pain is a common symptom seeking explanation. The term 'arthritis' means joint pain. It is important to ascertain from the parents of a child with limb pain its periodicity, precipitating and relieving events, and most importantly, whether or not they have noticed any swelling or redness in the affected part.

All students must be able to examine all joints, but particularly (a) the hand (b) the hip and (c) the knee, these being the joints most commonly involved in arthritic process.

Joint examination

Correct examination of any joint depends upon:
- inspection and accurate description of observations
- palpation for heat, tenderness, swelling, and crepitus
- testing range of movement.

Joint inspection involves looking for the presence of joint swelling, for loss of usual bony landmarks and joint contours, and for associated muscle wasting. In the knee, wrist and interphalangeal joints, swelling may be obvious. Swollen interphalangeal joints produce a spindle-shaped deformity of the finger. Swelling of the wrist joint may result in a 'dinner-fork' deformity of the hand.

Joint palpation implies a search for joint heat using the palm side or back of one's hand according to preference. One must compare joints with one another and with surrounding structures. Joint tenderness may be assessed by gently pressing, compressing or squeezing the joint. It may be important to decide if joint swelling is due to synovial thickening, or to the presence of fluid, or both. Fluid in the knee joint is indicated by a positive patellar tap.

Joint movement requires a knowledge of the normal range of movement of a given joint (about 180° at the wrist and 140° at the knee, for example) and an insistence that active movements always be performed prior to passive movements.

Arthritis

This is manifest by the presence of the classical signs of inflammation:

- rubor (redness)
- calor (heat)
- dolor (pain)
- tumour (swelling), and
- functiolasia (loss of function).

The term juvenile chronic arthritis (JCA) is now used to describe the various chronic arthritides of childhood. Below is a proposed classification of JCA.

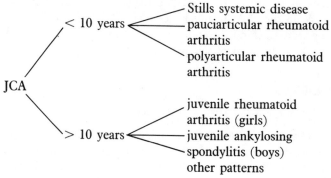

JCA

< 10 years
— Stills systemic disease
— pauciarticular rheumatoid arthritis
— polyarticular rheumatoid arthritis

> 10 years
— juvenile rheumatoid arthritis (girls)
— juvenile ankylosing spondylitis (boys)
— other patterns

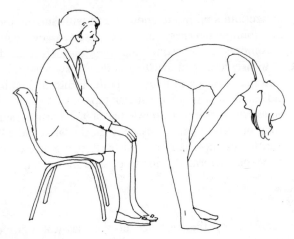

Fig. 5.17 Inspecting for scoliosis.

Scoliosis

Routine examination, particularly in adolescent schoolgirls, should include inspection for scoliosis. Scoliosis is sought by:
1. Inspection from behind in the upright posture. One shoulder may be elevated and the lumbar or thoracic spine may apparently be curved. It is usual to describe the curvature on the basis of its convexity (to right or left).
2. Asking the child to touch her toes. The examiner should be seated behind the child with eyes horizontal to the bent back. A fixed socoliosis will be evidenced by a hump.

THE EYES

  'The eye is the window of the soul'.

The eyes can tell a lot about all of us. When indulging in the art of physiognomy (attempting to assess character from facial features) one first looks at the eyes. So too in children. The dull, sunken eyes in dehydration; the sad, depressed eyes in marasmic malnutrition; the yellow sclera of jaundice; the pink iris of albinism; the bright, sparkling eyes of gaiety and good health.

Eye examination should include:
- general inspection of the eye, pupil, iris, sclera
- assessment of eye movement, with a comment on symmetry or otherwise
- pupillary, accommodation and corneal reflexes as appropriate
- red reflex
- retinal fundoscopy (with the ophthalmoscope)
- assessment of visual acuity.

Ophthalmoscopy

Good ophthalmoscopy is an integral part of examination of any child, irrespective of age. In the newborn, assistance is required to hold the head correctly in the midline. The eyelids can be gently prised apart. Elicit the red reflex in both eyes from a distance of 20 cm. Inspect the cornea for clarity, seek any lens opacity, and examine the fundus to detect haemorrhages, retinopathy and appearance of the disc.

Fundoscopy can be very difficult in toddlers and preschool children. Keep the infant or child in his position of comfort — lying, sitting on his mother's knee, or sitting alone. Darken the room if necessary. Keep the light intensity of the ophthalmoscope down. Do not use mydriatics (without permission). Try to get the child to look at an attractive but distracting object. Do not force the eyes open — this usually results in resistance and rejection. Be patient, approaching slowly from a distance. Patience and perseverance may be rewarded by the recognition of an identifiable retinopathy (for example rubella, cytomegalovirus or toxoplasma retinopathy in a child whose handicaps were previously unexplained).

Other rare findings include: retinopathy of prematurity

('retrolental fibroplasia'), hypertensive retinopathy, choroidal tubercle, toxocara (ocular larva migrans). Papilloedema is very rare in the presence of open fontanelle and sutures.

Fundoscopy findings

- rubella retinopathy: = 'pepper and salt' appearance on retina
- toxoplasmosis: = one or many pigmented or atrophic scars
- cherry red spot: = seen in a variety of rare inherited disorders.

In infants and children always first ask the mother: Does your child see well? If she replies yes, ask her to tell you her reasons. She's usually right. If she thinks her child sees poorly, seek the reason. The onus lies on the doctor to determine whether she's right or wrong.

Occasional eye findings of no consequence

1. *Pseudostrabismus* (pseudosquint) is the spurious appearance of a squint due to broad nasal bridge or prominent epicanthic folds.
2. *Blue sclera* are usually normal in infancy. Strikingly blue sclerae are seen in osteogenesis imperfecta and in inherited connective tissue disorders.
3. *Blinking* is often a form of habit spasm or tic in schoolchildren, best ignored.
4. *Light reflection* is useful at all ages. Light from a distant source (the window, a light bulb, or torch) should fall symmetrically on the pupils through all range of movements.

Normal values for ocular landmarks (Fig. 5.19) can be

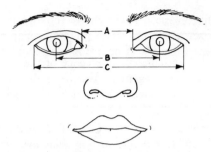

Fig. 5.18 Ocular landmarks: A = intercanthal distance B = interpupillary distance C = outer canthal distance.

found in specialized texts. Hypertelorism exists when the eyes are widely spaced apart.

The term 'mongoloid slant' is used when the eyes slope upwards and outward. By converse, 'anti-mongoloid slant' is downward and outward.

Observational ophthalmology

We have stressed throughout this text the rewards of careful observation. A good look at the eyes is well worthwhile:

1. *Cataract* may be seen. Cataracts are associated with congenital rubella and galactosaemia.
2. *Corneal clouding* may be apparent. This is suggestive of mucopolysacchoidosis.
3. *Nystagmus* may be noted.
4. Roving, purposeless eye movements with little visual fixation are typical of the infant with visual impairment.
5. *Ptosis* of the eyelid may be obvious.
6. Males with the fragile X syndrome have cold (often blue) piercing eyes.
7. The 'frozen watchfulness' of the battered or abused child may be observed. His gaze is calculated and seems to go through you.

Come to terms: eyes

amblyopia	= 'lazy' eye; partial loss of vision
aniridia	= congenital absence of the iris
anophthalmia	= congenital absence of the eye (orbit)
aphakia	= congenital absence of the lens

A few simple points to remember about eye examination are that children do not like having their eyes prised open, that accommodation is strong in preschool children, that pupillary inequality is an occasional normal finding, and that symmetry of movement, colour, and reaction is important to establish.

Eye examination at different ages

Newborn

Newborn infants dislike strong light; however, turning to light is a useful clinical test during the first month. Transitory fixation may be elicited by bringing a red (ball) object into the visual field at a distance of about 30–50 cm.

The newborn's eyes are best examined with the baby upright, and, if necessary, sucking. They will usually open in this position. With patience and a co-operative baby you may see the baby's eyes 'lock' onto his mother's.

At birth, examination is mainly to exclude gross abnormalities, evidence of possible trauma and congenital or acquired infection. Eye movement at this stage is established through the use of the vestibular ocular reflex, where rotating the infant from side to side, backwards and forwards and up and down, will elicit eye movements in all directions.

Disconjugate movements may be present in the first week or two but are usually gone by 4 weeks. Eye size should be checked to exclude eyes that are too big (glaucoma) or too small (microphthalmia). The cornea should be perfectly clear within one to two days after birth. The pupils should be equal and reactive. Always be suspicious of different coloured eyes at this stage. Assessment of alignment is best carried out with an ophthalmoscope at about a distance of 0.5 m. At this distance the examiner can observe both pupils simultaneously and compare redness and brightness of the red reflex. If inequality of the redness occurs, the possibility of a strabismus or an opacity in the eye should be considered. Fundoscopy at this stage shows occasional haemorrhages particularly around the disc and posterior pole. If the haemorrhages are extensive, an ophthalmological opinion should be sought. Sometimes in the first few days, oedema of the eyelids causes difficulty in opening the eye for proper examination and in this case placing the infant in the prone position will facilitate eye opening.

6–8 weeks

The infant is alert to moving objects although convergence and following are jerky. An examiner can readily hold the infant's attention at a distance of about 30 cm and a rewarding smile 'with meaning' is elicited. By 12 weeks head and eye movements may be demonstrated through 180°. At this age lacrimal glands will show response to emotion.

16–20 weeks

Hand regard develops and a 1 inch brick will cause immediate fixation within a distance of 1 m. Colour preference develops from 20–28 weeks and hand/eye co-ordination (palmar grasp) can readily be elicited using brick or paper. Visual acuity continues to improve dramatically from 9 to 12 months and very small objects can be seen and picked up using index finger and thumb. There is smooth visual movement in both the horizontal and vertical planes. At 1 year the transverse diameter of the cornea is adult size (12 mm). Convergence is well established by 18 months. By the age of 4 years visual acuity is nearly 20/20.

Examination of the eyes should be carried out in every patient irrespective of age. Skill in the proper use of the ophthalmoscope should be acquired early in clinical training. Assessment should occur in the neonatal period, at the toddler stage (2–3 years) and again at 5 years (preschool). Subsequently to this, assessment should be carried out every 2–3 years to late teens.

Strabismus (squint)

Parents will often offer the opinion that their child has a squint. Squint may be more apparent when the child is tired. Relatives or friends may point out a squint to the parents. Students should always accept parents' opinion concerning squint and test the eyes appropriately. Squint in the newborn is not significant so long as you can exclude a retinoblastoma. Approach squints in the following fashion:

1. Look for light reflection through all movements.
2. Test eye movement and muscles in all directions.
3. Try to answer the simple question — is this squint alternating (concomitant) or paralytic?
4. Look for corneal opacities and cataracts.
5. Do the *cover test*. Use an interesting object (toy) to hold the child's attention. The eye is covered on the visual axis to make viewing of the object monocular. If the child has been fixing with the eye just covered, the other eye will take over fixation in the presence of a squint.

Any squint persisting beyond 5–6 months from birth is significant and should be referred immediately to an ophthalmologist. Pseudosquint is a common minor variation. Paralytic squint, though rare, tends to have more serious connotations than alternating squint.

The red reflex

Shine a light at both eyes from a distance of 0.5 m. There should be a symmetrical red reflex. A white pupillary reflex will be caused by cataract, retinoblastoma and retinopathy of prematurity. Absence of the red reflex is called leukocoria.

Come to terms: eye lumps

chalazion	= small inclusion cyst in eyelid
hordeolum	= stye in the eye (pustule)
dermoid	= external angle dermoid of eye
pinguecula	= small yellowish patch near the cornea

Occasional eye findings

1. *Dilated* conjunctival vessels may suggest ataxia — telangiectasia.
2. *Brushfield's spots* (white spots around the outer iris) are seen in Down's syndrome but also in normal children.
3. *Morgan-Dennie fold* is a double fold under the eye. It is seen in eczematous, allergic children.

The neurological examination and interpretation of the eyes are similar in children and adults. Pupils should normally be equal, central, circular and respond to light and accommodation. Eye movements should be full in all directions. Fine nystagmus on extreme deviation is a normal finding. The corneal reflex is unpleasant and rarely needs to be elicited. We will not detail testing of visual acuity at different ages — refer to Mary Sheridan's book (1975) or to a textbook of ophthalmology. In co-operative children, visual fields can be roughly assessed by confrontation tests.

In early infancy the following may be warning signs of *poor visual acuity*:

- roving or wandering eye movements

- persistence of hand regard
- lack of blink to a hand thrust rapidly toward the face ('blinking to menace')
- nystagmus.

Early detection and treatment of squint can prevent amblyopia. Early detection of reduced visual acuity can lead to appropriate therapy.

At all clinic visits ask the mother:

Can your baby see well?

Tell me why you think so.

If she's worried about her baby's vision take her on her word. Her insight is usually right!

6

A measure of progress

'A paediatrician is a measuring doctor'

Apley

Chesterton has stated that the man who knew him best was his tailor, for he measured him afresh each time he met him. The same should be said of children's doctors, who should habitually measure length (height), weight and head circumference of all infants and toddlers. In addition, arm circumference, skinfold thickness, blood pressure, upper-lower segment ratios, etc., will be measured as appropriate.

In infancy, lying length is measured. Most crudely this can be done by measuring crown-heel length using a tape. More accurate methods are horizontal stadiometers or the 'pedo-baby' measurer. Standing *height* can be measured against simple wall charts, against vertical rulers, or using a stadiometer. The most accurate methods have been established by Tanner's group. Buckler's text (1979) is full of useful tables, graphs, charts and information. Height should ideally be plotted on a centile chart appropriate for sex, age and race. In early age (up to 7 years) there is little sex difference. International charts have been published. Height increment is probably a better indicator of well-being than weight gain.

It has been said in the Bible that a just *weight* is the Lord's delight and a false balance an abomination; so too in paediatrics. All babies, infants and toddlers need to be weighed regularly. Drug dosages and fluid requirements are related to body weight. In the first year of life, weight will increase threefold, length by 50% and head circumference by approximately one-third.

Head circumference, or more correctly, maximal occipitofrontal diameter, should also be measured using a non-stretchable and reliable tape. Head circumference is an indicator of brain growth (but not of intelligence). One is looking for heads which are growing unusually rapidly or unusually slowly. In ordinary practice one usually defines the upper and lower third centiles (which are equivalent to ±2 SD) as the borders of 'normality'. Measurements less than the third centile do not necessarily imply abnormality: many of these will be 'small normals'.

Height and head circumference, for example, do run in families. Cognizance of parents' height must always be taken in assessment of short stature. Charts for equating children's height with mid-parental height are available. Familial macrocephaly is a well recognized entity — parental head circumference measurement is an essential part of the assessment of any infant or child with an unusually large head.

Other useful measurement include:

1. *Arm span*: from fingertip to fingertip, across shoulders. This should approximate standing height from age 3–4 years. If less than height it may suggest short limbs.
2. *Upper-lower segment ratio*: the measurements are from pubis to crown, and from pubis to ground. In the schoolchild the ratio is close to unity. It is 1.7 : 1 in the newborn.
3. *Arm circumference*: halfway between the shoulder and the elbow. In developing countries this is a useful index of nutrition.
4. *Skinfold thickness*: using an appropriate caliper. Measurement usually made in the left mid-tripces region and in the left subcapular area. These are used to gauge under and overnutrition.

5. Height (and weight) *velocity* which measures the rate of change as opposed to the distance achieved.

Somebody has measured just about everything imaginable relating to children — interpupillary distance, stretched penile length, testicular volume, kidney size, cardiothoracic ratio — and their normal values can be obtained from specialized texts.

- plot on centile charts
- serial measurements more important than single ones
- patterns of aberrant growth are well recognized
- children tend to stick to centile channels.

In approaching the unusually small or tall child, simple questions, accurate measurements and appropriate centile and velocity chartings will often save a lot of time and much unnecessary investigation. A typical algorithm for approaching the small child is shown below.

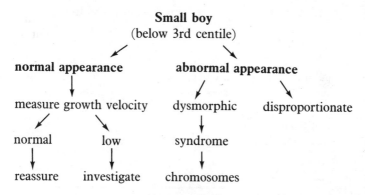

Small boy
(below 3rd centile)

normal appearance   **abnormal appearance**

measure growth velocity   dysmorphic   disproportionate

normal   low   syndrome

reassure   investigate   chromosomes

If there are no previous measurements on a small child, his mother should be asked about shoe size, clothes size and age (many large stores label clothes by age), and you could ask to inspect family photographs. While doctors may be concerned about a small child, his mother may be nonplussed since 'all my family were slow starters'.

Children, especially boys, are conscious of their height and earnestly wish to match their peers. We don't entirely agree with the 'bottom line' in the following little poem:

> I met a little Elfman once,
> Down where the lilies blow,
> I asked him why he was so small,
> And why he did not grow.
> He slightly frowned and with his eyes,
> He looked me through and through,
> 'I'm quite as big for me, he said,
> As you are big for you'.

John K. Bangs

Finally, some simple pointers:

- centile charts describe what is, not what should be
- there may be a significant difference in height between the best and worse off segments in society, but not necessarily in weight
- most small children are 'small normal' children coming from families of small parents and/or from socially deprived groups
- there is probably nothing wrong with those small children (below third centile) who demonstrate normal growth velocity observed over 6–12 months
- static height or weight in a child is unusual and may be a sign of disease
- crossing down centile channels is abnormal.

Come to terms: short stature

diastrophic dwarfism	= crooked dwarfism
thanatophoric dwarfism	= death bearing dwarfism
achondroplasia	= a form of short-limbed dwarfism
osteopetrosis	= marble bone disease

We believe that students need not spend too much time on rare and unusual cases, however interesting they may be. If you can stimulate the skill of recognizing what's different, if you can describe what you see, and if you know suitable sources of further information, that should suffice.

Dysmorphology depends on recognition, description and measurement. One can consult appropriate texts or a suitably programmed computer.

The *measurements used in dysmorphology* include:

- height
- arm span
- upper-lower segment ratios
- hand length
- metacarpal length
- ear length
- interocular distance
- forearm carrying angle
- inner canthal distance
- bone age.

7

Hydration and nutrition

DETECTING AND DETERMINING DEHYDRATION

In maintaining normal hydration infants are dependent on their attendants (mother, nurse, etc) to supply a sufficient quantity of fluid. For a variety of physiological and practical reasons, dehydration can arise easily and rapidly in infancy. Early detection and determination of the degree of dehydration is therefore essential.

Why is dehydration common in infants?

1. Infants have a different body composition to adults — 70–80% body water content versus 60% in adults.
2. High fluid intake — 150 ml/kg/day compared to 30–40 ml/kg/day in adults.
3. Daily water turnover of 10–15% of body weight compared to 3–5% in adults.
4. Relative reduction in renal ability to concentrate urine.
5. Greater surface area/mass ratio resulting in high insensible fluid losses through skin and respiratory tract. Factor X2–3.
6. Higher basal metabolic rate plus greater febrile response to infection.
7. Infants have little or no control over fluid intake.

A normal state of hydration is manifest by bright eyes, moist tongue and good skin turgor. Fat infants (in whom skin

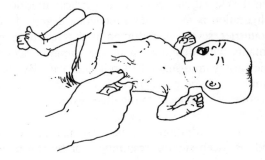

Fig. 7.1 Loss of normal skin turgor.

turgor is difficult to determine) may deceive by concealing dehydration, especially of the hypertonic type. Appreciation of normal skin turgor or elasticity is best established by examining lots of normal infants.

Signs of dehydration

Dehydration in infancy is manifested by:
1. A sunken anterior fontanelle.
2. Dull, dry eyes with reduced eyeball turgor (as most of us do not normally assess eyeball turgor in normal infants, one can be uncertain of this sign).
3. Dry tongue and mouth.
4. Diminished skin turgor or elasticity, which is best elicited by picking up abdominal or thigh skin.
5. Lethargy and weak cry.
6. Diminished pulse volume.
7. Diminished urinary output (more dry nappies).
8. Reduced blood pressure.

It is important to remember that the early signs of dehydration reflect loss of interstitial fluid volume whereas the later signs (6–8) reflect loss of intravascular volume. Most infants in developed countries get to medical attention when their dehydration is of a mild to moderate degree. In developing countries severe dehydration is a frequent phenomenon. Infants with dehydration of the common isotonic or hypotonic variety are usually lethargic and 'flat'. By contrast, hyperteronic or hypernatraemic dehydration, which introduces a cerebral component to the illnesses, may be suspected if the infant is irritable or cranky.

Very severe dehydration may be accompanied by a metabolic acidosis (deep sighing respiration) or by shock (pallid, cold, quiet infant).

Fluid facts

	1 week	1 year	20 years
Weight (kg)	3.0	10.0	70.0
Length (cm)	50	75	175
Head circumference (cm)	35	46	55
Body surface area (m²)	0.25	0.5	1.73
Blood pressure (mmHg)	70/40	90/50	120/80
Fluid intake (l/day)	0.45	1.0	2.5
Fluid intake (% BW)	15	10	3.5
Fluid intake (ml/kg/day)	150	100	35

The figures in the table highlight the important differences in fluid balance between the neonate, infant and adult. It must be emphasized that these are 'typical' values and that there is much variation.

Types of dehydration

- isotonic: (70%) flat, lethargic
- hypotonic: (20–30%)
- hypertonic: (2–5%) irritable, 'doughy' skin, convulsions.

It can be difficult to clinically determine the type of dehydration. It is important to be alert and to try to detect hypertonic dehydration, as this may result in convulsions and brain damage.

The degree of dehydration

- mild (0–5% loss of body weight) = few clinical signs. Perhaps dry tongue, flattish fontanelle
- moderate (5–10% loss of body weight) = obvious clinical signs of loss of interstitial fluid — sunken fontanelle, dry tongue, reduced skin turgor
- severe (10–15% loss of body weight) = seriously ill. Signs of loss of intravascular volume — weak, fast pulse, low blood pressure, poor urine output — plus earlier signs.

Mild — moderate dehydra- = ↓ interstitial volume
tion
Severe dehydration = ↓ intravascular volume

Overhydration is less frequently encountered in children but may occur with cardiac faillure, renal failure or excessive intravenous fluids. One might clinically attempt to estimate the degree of fluid overload (weight increase as a proportion of dry weight, if known) and aim to restore water balance by fluid restriction, diuretics or dialysis as appropriate. The cardinal clinical sign is oedema.

NUTRITION

Clinical assessment of nutrition is relatively simple. Modern western infant malnutrition consists of children being fed the wrong foods (too much carbohydrate) and too many calories, resulting in obesity. In the developing world, protein, calorie, vitamin and mineral deficiencies are common. Inadequate food intake is a common cause of failure to thrive in all parts of the world.

Assessment of nutrition

- look
- weigh, measure and plot on centile chart
- examination for specific deficiencies.

Observation

The well infant has full cheeks, firm rounded buttocks, good muscle tone and a healthy complexion. Acute malnutrition in infancy manifests as weight loss, loose subcutaneous skin folds, and apathy. Chronic malnutrition is evidenced by pallor, thinness, prominent bones, protuberant abdomen, hypotonia, flat buttocks and misery. The skin may be thin and shiny, the hair dull and lack lustre, and the nails brittle.

Weighing and measuring

This has been described in Chapter 6. Remember that centile charts describe what is, not what should be. They are gathered from normal children in a given population. Many of the children in the upper 'normal' centile ranges in western populations look fat — they *are* fat.

Watch carefully those children who are crossing down centile lines.

The 'normal' thin child tends to have similar parents, to be active and sturdy, and to have proportionate height and weight centiles.

Growth is probably a better indicator of well-being than weight. Significant differences in height exist between the upper and lower social groups in most populations: weight differences may not be so evident.

Examination for specific deficiencies

Iron deficiency is the commonest type.

Anaemia: Inspect conjunctival mucous membrane, buccal mucous membrane, palmar creases and nailbeds for redness, or pallor. Iron-deficient children are frequently unhappy or miserable. In Caucasian children facial pallor is more often a matter of skin complexion and lack of sunlight than of anaemia. However, healthy babies do have a good pink complexion.

Rickets is due to vitamin D deficiency and is manifest by limb pain, widening of wrist bones, knock knees, and the 'rickety rosary'. The 'rickety rosary' is caused by expansion of the costochondral junctions, which are more lateral than many students think.

Protein: severe protein deficiency is seen in kwashiorkor. The child so affected is apathetic, has flaky skin, reddish thin hair, and oedema of face or legs.

Folic acid, vitamin B_{12} and vitamin C deficiency are all rare in western children. However, scurvy and other vitamin deficiencies may be seen in children fed on strict vegetarian ('vegan') diets.

8

Developmental assessment

Developmental assessment is an integral part of paediatrics and it is essential that normal development is well understood. Know the norm and the many variations thereof. In general terms, it is accepted that the most appropriate ages for assessment are 6–8 weeks (described elsewhere), 6 months, 9–10 months, 18 months, 2 years, and finally at 4–5 years, prior to school entry.

It is of the utmost importance to have a detailed perinatal history and in particular an adverse one. There are many textbooks on the subject of developmental paediatrics and all give guidelines to examination which is based on the assessment of gross motor, vision and fine motor, hearing and speech and social behaviour. Each of these are interdependent and complementary. However it is most helpful to try to isolate an area of delay.

At 12 weeks:
- lies back with head in midline
- waves hands symmetrically and brings into midline
- head erect and steady — to 30°
- lifts head and upper chest in prone position
- hand regard.

Having assessed the 6 to 8-week-old previously, usually the next assessment is from 6–9 months. However, significant changes are occuring in the interval between 2 and 6 months. Most primitive reflexes preseent at birth, should be entirely absent from 4 months. If present after this time, this suggests that the brain is not developing in line with chronological age either as a result of a generalized brain disorder or a specific lesion giving rise to pyramidal tract lesions. Gross motor achievements at this time include sophisticated head control, attempting to roll over, and sitting aided. Convergence is complete and visual acuity is improving, and hands are reaching to attempt grasp. The baby responds to but does not turn to sound. Babbling is well established. Social development reflects a well nourished, alert, confident and secure child. Tragically, social and environmental problems can detrimentally impinge at an early age.

It must be stressed that at any developmental assessment examination both mother and baby should be put at ease and made comfortable. Initial discussion should concern the previous history and inquiry into the general behaviour of the infant to date should be made. Complementary remarks about baby to mother are helpful. Under no circumstances should one initially attempt physical examination. Sit, watch, observe, particularly the size, disposition, appearance and general demeanour of your patient.

- Remember, social deprivation may influence adversely at an early age.

6 TO 8 MONTHS

Normal gross motor development at this time will include sitting without support, rolling over and the ability to extend the arms and lift the chest in the prone position. Lateral righting and parachute reflexes are becoming established and sophisticated.

Visual acuity can now be reasonably well assessed using the methods described by Sheridan (1975). At a distance of 3 m a selection of white balls down to 2 cm will be followed. Eye movement can also be commented on. Strabismus is significant at this age. Improving visual acuity allows for significant development of hand/eye co-ordination where an infant can reach out and with palmar grasp and retrieve a small object (brick) which will be examined, probably transferred to the other hand and finally put to the mouth. Usually hand dominance is not established at this time. The infant at this age will also turn to sound at a distance of 0.5 m in a horizontal line from the ear. It is often noted that around 5–6 months one ear may respond better than the other. Enhanced response usually occurs in the ear addressed by the nursing mother. The sounds used as stimulus include the speech frequencies (500–2000 Hz) with crumpled paper, rattle, and cup and spoon. Socially, the infant is usually happy with strangers, laughs easily, will respond to talking and will be babbling more precisely, that is, 'dada' and 'baba'.

6 months

— *Motor*
  - good head control
  - rolls over
  - sits momentarily
  - back straight.
— *Vision and fine movement*
  - alert
  - eyes move in all directions
  - fixates on small object — 20 cm
  - palmar grasp — transfer.
— *Hearing and speech*
  - turns to sound 0.5 m
  - mothers voice discerned
  - vocalizes — Ka, Dah.
— *Social*
  - takes everything to mouth

- tries to hold bottle
- can elicit noise from rattle
- responds to tickling.
— **Warnings**
  - maternal anxiety
  - head circumference less than 3rd centile
  - hypotonia — poor head control
  - hypertonia — brisk reflexes and clonus
  - not alert— failure to fixate or strabismus
  - not turning to sound (beware unilateral response)
  - persistent primitive reflexes.

9 TO 10 MONTHS

— *Motor*
  - sits alone and can turn to look
  - can move on floor — rolling, squirming, crawling
  - will support weight when upright and will probably hold on
  - does not like being moved from sitting to lying supine
  - protective reflexes well established.
— *Vision and fine movement*
  - very observant
  - pincer grasp with good manipulation
  - looks after fallen toy
  - can see small object at 3 m.
— *Hearing and speech*
  - may know and turn to name
  - test hearing at 1 m
  - babbles loudly and incessantly.
— *Social*
  - holds, bites and chews biscuit
  - grasps bottle when feeding
  - beginning of suspicion of strangers

10 months

— **Warnings**.
- maternal anxiety
- head circumference < 3rd centile
- not sitting
- poor protective reflexes
- asymmetry of tone
- brisk reflexes or clonus
- poor vocalization
- poor response to sound
- unable to chew.

12 MONTHS

At 12 months there may be considerable variation in developmental status particularly in gross motor. At this time the infant should be sitting and turning without difficulty. Most will be crawling or have a variation thereof to include rolling over, bottom shuffling, sidestroking and bear walk (back legs extended). Standing with or without support should be achieved, some will walk holding on or on their own. In general terms if an infant walks into the examination room aged 1 year, you can almost turn him around and walk him out again.

Visual acuity has improved and a 1 cm diameter ball is followed at 3 m. Objects are now picked up, using the more sophisticated thumb-index finger or pincer grasp. Objects receive more attention and examination. However they still reach the mouth. The baby will search for an object falling from view. The sound frequencies used for the 6-month-old are now applied at a distance of 1 m from the ear and in a 180° arc at each side. Vocabulary has improved both in pronunciation and number of words (2–3). The infant comprehends simple commands — wave 'day-day', clap hands. Socially the infant is now wary of strangers and makes strange and clings to his mother. However, he responds to his own name, and plays purposefully with toys.

At this age major areas of delay should have surfaced to include — poor brain growth, gross motor delay, visual and hearing impairment and in particular, cerebral palsy of the spastic type. Even at this early age, prognostic projections are possible.

18 MONTHS

— *Motor*
- walks
- may run — straight
- creeps backwards downstairs
- picks up toy from floor without falling.

— *Vision and fine movement*
- builds 2–3 bricks
- points to distant objects (outside)
- hand preference appearing
- shows distinct interest in human face.

— *Hearing and language*
- vocalizes freely
- up to 20 words
- responds quickly to simple commands.

— *Social*
- drinks without spilling
- hands cup back to adult
- has stopped putting toys into mouth.

— **Warnings**
- maternal anxiety
- not standing
- not walking
- poor attention span.

Developmental assessment is an integral part of every clinic visit. We would hope that accurate developmental examination will facilitate early detection of problems. We have itemized early warning signals, which make specialized referral mandatory. We would refer you to specialized texts for follow-on examinations at older ages.

Note. The rate of development may vary between children. The sequence of development does not differ significantly. Loss of primitive reflexes is paralleled by a gain of positive skills.

Developmental decisions
- normal
- probably normal — see again
- doubtful — see again *soon*
- abnormal — refer for diagnosis and treatment.

Some commentators prefer the term developmental 'stepping stones' to developmental 'milestones'. Remember that whatever term you use, development is about progress and change. Described below are some locomotion variants to give appreciation of the range of normality.

Locomotion variants
- Some infants never crawl; they stand and walk
- some do normal crawl with flexed knees
- some do sidestroke (swing) crawl
- some do bear walk (knees extended)
- some roll from A to B
- some bounce around floor on bottom.

9

Examining excreta

THE STOOL MEDICAL INSPECTION

Paediatric ward sisters often rightly complain of the lack of interest shown by junior medical staff or students in stools. One wonders how some doctors know what are abnormal stools since they know so little of what is normal. Even when presented suitably wrapped in transparent film and appropriately perfumed, stools are unwillingly examined or observed with haste and distaste.

What is normal stool frequency, consistency, colour, odour? This is determined by feeding contents and pattern. The experienced ward sister knows, of course, that certain conditions can display characteristic stools discernible at a glance. While the descriptions given below are 'classic' examples of certain conditions, recognizable patterns in stool passage and stool appearance amongst infants may direct one down an appropriate diagnostic pathway. When it comes to children's stool medical inspection, listen carefully to the mother's description and the ward sister's interpretation. Also remember that the stools may be apparently 'normal' in proven coeliac disease or cystic fibrosis.

Breast fed motions. These are soft, bright yellow (like scrambled eggs) with a fragrant acid odour. Frequency can vary from 3–6 per day. Volume is usually less than formula motions.

Formula fed motions are usually more formed than breast fed stools, will vary from brown to yellowish to a powdery green. Some proprietary formulae do produce characteristic stools.

Hunger stools are not now often seen in Western countries. They are traditionally described as being like spinach, green, loose.

Coeliac disease. The typical stools are large, pale, bulky and offensive. A normal stool pattern, or even constipation, does not exclude coeliac disease.

Cystic fibrosis. The motions are bulky, greasy, and singularly offensive. But are not all stools intrinsically offensive? Certainly. The mother of a child recently diagnosed of cystic fibrosis informed us 'you'd need a gas mask to change him'.

Toddler diarrhoea (irritable bowel of infancy). The motions are frequent (3–5 per day), messy ('they run down his leg, doctor'), brown, mucusy, and contain vegetable matter (especially peas, carrots, corn and tomatoes). The Americans aptly label this 'peas and carrots syndrome'.

Disaccharide intolerance. Frequent, watery, acidic ('they burn his bottom') stools often associated with the passage of flatus.

Acute gastroenteritis. Watery, green, frequent, offensive, poorly formed motions. Bloody diarrhoea may suggest a *Salmonella* or *Shigella* aetiology.

Liver disease. Motions may be pale.

Intussusception. Classical motions are described as being 'like redcurrant jelly'.

Iron. May darken the motions.

Rifampicin. May stain the motions an orange colour.

Worms. Threadworms, roundworms, tapeworms, and whipworms may be seen in freshly passed motions.

In conclusion, going through the motions is important in determining the cause of acute and chronic diarrhoeal diseases in children. The start of paediatric gastroenterology is to take oneself to stool examination.

CAST YOUR EYE ON THE URINE

While inspection of sputum, vomitus, or stools may be ignored by students (at their peril) examination of the urine cannot. Urine needs to be inspected, occasionally smelt, 'dipsticked' and subjected to light microscopy. It is beyond the scope of this book to discuss the causes of haematuria, or red urine ('haemastix' negative), or leucocyturia. But we do insist that students know how to interpret routine 'dipstick' analysis for protein, blood, ketones, etc., how to recognize red and white cells on unspun, unstained urine, and how to identify casts.

On the sideroom door in one London children's unit one used to read the notice: 'Richard Bright omitted to examine the urine with a microscope — you can do better'. (Richard Bright described glomerulonephritis in 1850, but eschewed the microscope).

Urine colour and concentration can be inspected. Orange urine is induced by jaundice and by rifampicin. The first sign of acute glomerulonephritis may be the passage of red, dark, tea or 'coke' coloured urine. Dilute watery urine may be seen in diabetes insipidus (central or nephrogenic) and in polydipsic states. The frothiness of albumen-containing urine was first noted in Hippocratic times.

The presence of granular or red cell casts in the urine is pathognomic of acute glomerulonephritis. Casts should be sought in any child with acute haematuria. With a little tuition and lots of looking students can come to recognize red cells, white cells and bacteria in unstained urine. Time spent peering down the microscope will be repaid in practice. Hyaline casts are a normal finding.

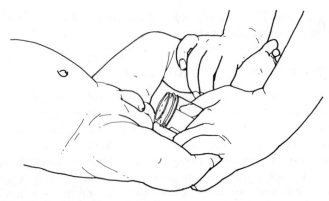

Fig. 9.1 Awaiting a clean catch urine.

Urine cloudiness is a common finding and may reflect the presence of dissolved chemicals (urates, phosphates) or of leucocytes. Dissolved urates will precipitate out on standing and the sediment frequently has a pinkish hue; this is a normal finding. The presence of leucocyturia suggests urinary tract infection.

One may occasionally see threadworm cysts in fresh urine.

Urine collection

AGE	METHODS	COMMENT
Infancy	Clean catch	Best; requires patience
Infancy	Bladder massage	See p. 42
Infancy	Bladder percussion	Sometimes works
Infancy, toddler	Bag	Remove quickly, avoid contamination
Toddler	Standing in bath	Useful way of getting MSU
Toilet trained child	Classical MSU	Best
Any	Catheter	Rarely necessary; avoid
Infant	Bladder stab	Acutely ill; failed MSU. Rarely necessary
Any	Running tap, cold water	Often works!

10

Using your senses

A CACOPHONY OF CRIES

> 'But what am I
> An infant crying in the night
> An infant crying for the light
> And with no language but a cry'

Tennyson

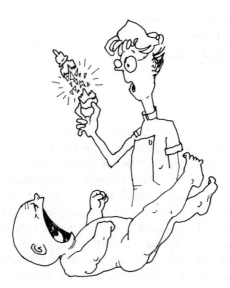

Fig. 10.1 Infant cry.

Probably the most important, relished, and long-awaited cry a child will make in his life is the first exclamatory cry he makes on emerging, relieved, from the birth canal.

The infant's ability to express himself is very limited, especially in his early days and months. The same symptoms — poor feeding, lethargy, vomiting, fever — may signal many different impending infections or illnesses. As such his cry is of crucial importance as a means of communication. His cry may be trying to tell you something.

Mothers soon get to know their baby's collection of 'normal' cries signifying hunger, wind, wet, dirty, or loneliness. Students too need to open their ears and listen.

A short period of nursing duties — feeding, changing, observing babies — is of considerable value to all students during their paediatric course. It cannot be said too often — you will not readily recognize the abnormal unless you are familiar with the normal.

We wish to refer briefly to:
- cries of pain
- cries of certain illnesses
- cries of some conditions.

Pain

Probably the most important cry to recognize is that of *pain* in infancy. The most alarming cry is that heard in association with meningitis, encephalitis, or raised intracranial pressure from whatever cause. Mothers will usually describe this as high-pitched, shrill, screeching, screaming or piercing. Always take note of the mother who says 'his cry has changed, it's different'. In addition to the particular cry, infants with intracranial lesions can be difficult to console. The cry which accompanies infantile spasms can be short, sharp, high-pitched and is not infrequently thought to be due to 'colic'. It is not unusual for a cry to accompany an epileptic seizure.

In short, the cry of pain is *different* from the infants usual cry and mother will usually detect this call. So listen to her.

Cries of illness

The cry of acute croup is hoarse. The cry of acute broncho-pneumonia may be weak and grunting. The cry of the infant with acute intussusception may be sudden and grunting. The severely ill infant has a weak, whimpering cry.

Characteristic cries

Characteristic cries are described in certain conditions. Congenital hypothyroidism (hopefully soon an obsolete condition with extension of screening) is associated with a hoarse, croaky cry. Once heard, the extraordinary mewling of the cri-du-chat syndrome is never forgotten. Crowing cry may indicate laryngomalacia or other laryngeal lesion.

All babies cry. It is normal to cry. Don't forget the baby who 'never cries' — he is not normal; one might suspect developmental delay with such a description.

A SENSE OF DIAGNOSIS

Most of us are well trained in using our eyes, hands and ears in aiding diagnosis but often unskilled in the remaining two senses, those of taste and smell. Some brief examples:
- phenylketonuria — 'mousy' smell from urine
- diabetic ketoacidosis — acetone on breath
- maple syrup urine disease — smell of fresh maple sap from urine
- fishy urine — ? proteus infection
- salty taste on kissing — may suggest cystic fibrosis.

THE DIAGNOSTIC TOUCH

At various parts of this text we have emphasized the importance of inspection and palpation in paediatric physical examination.

Teach the back of or ulnar border of your hand to detect
changes in temperature. Always palpate rashes. (see p. 113).
Allow your finger pulps the experience of palpating little
pulses in head, hands, and feet of infants.

THE LAST WORD

This text will have failed in its primary objectives if students
merely read it and fail to apply the principles. It is very
difficult to learn how to drive a car or to operate a computer
from the manual. So go to it, and examine as many children
as will allow you!

Appendices

1. Normal findings

1. Telangiectasia (spider naevi) on hands or face of children. One to three telangiectasia is a frequent finding in school-children.
2. Café-au-lait spots — a few scattered. More than six larger than 1.5 cm in diameter is suggestive of neurofibromatosis.
3. Lymph nodes — scattered, small, shotty nodes (see p. 100)
4. Innocent (physiological, flow) murmurs. Very common.
5. Stork-beak marks (capillary haemangiomata) on forehead and nape of neck.
6. Epstein's (epithelial) pearls on roof of mouth.
7. Slight breast swelling in male and female infants.
8. Sacrococcygeal pits and dimples.
9. Mongolian blue spots in African/Asian infants and in infants of mixed parentage.
10. Sinus arrhythmia.
11. Periodic breathing (in premature neonates but *not* in infancy)
12. Acrocyanosis (peripheral cyanosis) in newborn.
13. Forehead bruises on toddlers who have recently acquired the skill of walking.
14. Mild bowleggedness in toddlers.

15. Bruises (as many as 10–20) on knees and shins of active toddlers and preschool children.
16. Blue sclera in infants.
17. Single transverse palmar crease — in up to 5% of people.

2. Tools of the trade

1. Stethoscope, preferably with 'paediatric' bell and diaphragm.
2. Tape measure, preferably steel or disposable. Plastic tapes may stretch if boiled.
3. Appropriate centile charts for children of various ages, sex.
4. Sphygmomanometer — with a selection of cuff widths.
5. Auriscope with ear pieces of varying size. Use the largest ear piece which fits comfortably. A piece of rubber tubing to apply suction may be useful.
6. A good light source for examining the fauces.
7. An ophthalmoscope. Remember that children dislike bright lights shone in their eyes. Keep light intensity down.
8. A pencil and paper — to allow the child to write or draw when you're talking to his mother.
9. A selection of picture and reading books (as in the 'Ladybird' series).
10. A few toys.
11. Some bricks.
12. A mirror.
13. A rattle.
14. A bell.
15. Magnifying glass for looking at skin lesions.

Plus (if possible) 'the same kind, beaming smile that children could warm their hands at' (J. M. Barrie)

Some departments of child health will have simulators, on which useful experience and practice may be obtained without distressing or harming anyone. Some examples:

1. Baby-hippy, Medical Plastics, Chicago.
2. Resusci-baby, Laerdal, Norway.
3. Ophthalmoscopy mannequin, Ophthalmic Development Lab., Iowa, USA.

3. Tricks of the trade

1. Listening over the nose with a stethoscope (see p. 104).
2. Distraction techniques (see p. 26).
3. Use of the thumbs to palpate pulses is permissible (if not desirable). Some may better be able to fix and palpate femoral pulses of the wriggling infant with the thumbs than with the finger pulps.
4. Palpating over the child's hands in assessing abdominal pain or tenderness (see p. 30).
5. Use of the stethoscope to gauge doubtful abdominal 'tenderness' (see p. 30).
6. The auriscope is best held in a penhold grip — you are less likely to hurt the child (see p. 102).
7. Use of auriscope to look up noses (for foreign bodies).
8. To get a newborn infant to open his eyes, hold him upright, or give him something to suck (see p. 142). Don't try to prise the eyes open — it just doesn't work.
9. When assessing plagiocephaly (parallelogram skull) place a finger in each auditory canal and compare their relative positions (see p. 38).
10. Asking children to point to the site of the pain (see p. 29).
11. When looking at the throat ask the child to make a big yawn (see p. 105).
12. Keep preschool and playschool children on their feet for

as much of the examination as possible — they feel much less threatened.

13. Flatter children on how good they are, on a nice dress or shirt, or tell him he's the boss in his family.

14. Strike up a rapport by talking at child level or discussing his television show (e.g. 'The Muppets').

15. If in doubt about undescended testes, examine the child while squatting on a chair (see p. 95).

4. Biological warning signals

1. The infant who loves (and licks) salt — has he a salt losing state, for example cystic fibrosis or a tubulopathy?

2. The toddler who throws away bread and biscuits. Could this suggest coeliac disease?

3. The child who hates soft drinks and sweets. Should you consider sucrase-isomaltase deficiency?

4. The child who drinks *anything* — he may have true diabetes insipidus. In addition, he will usually wake at night seeking drinks.

5. The child who objects to milk — give lactose intolerance or milk allergy a thought.

6. The child who lies down. He is ill. Sick children are like animals — they lie down when ill (without having to be told to do so) and get up when better.

7. Refusal or unwillingness to move a limb usually suggests something serious — a fracture or osteomyelitis, for example.

5. Clinical curios

1. *The allergic salute*. Children with allergic rhinitis frequently rub their nose vigorously with the palm of their hand.

2. *'Screwdriving'*. Agitated or upset infants have a character-

istic habit of rotating their hands in a screwdriving motion.

3. *Yawning*. In the newborn may be indicative of seizure activity.

4. *'Cracked pot note'* is the sound obtained on percussing the skull in infants with raised intracranial pressure.

5. *Foreign bodies* may end up in nostrils, ears, vaginas, as well as in stomachs and chests.

6. We have come to respect two symptoms in infants and toddlers — *limp* and *torticollis*. While limp has many causes, a lingering limp is a well recognized presentation of acute leukaemia. Acute torticollis is unusual in early childhood — consider posterior fossa tumour in the absence of other explanation.

7. Most *breath-holding episodes* terminate spontaneously. Some may, however, progress to 'pallid syncope' (a vaso-vagal episode) or even to 'reflex anoxic seizures'.

8. Lip smacking and cycling lower limb movements are involuntary episodes of contraction of groups of muscles. They occur usually in the first 48 hours of life and are associated with asphyxial encephalopathy.

6. Rules of thumb

1. All that wheezes is not asthma, but when recurrent usually is.

2. All that whoops is not pertussis, but most is. Adenovirus and parapertusis may produce a whoop.

3. The more widespread the pain, the less likely it is to be organic.

4. An infant who continues to feed may be ill, but not seriously so.

5. Viral infections tend to spread (ears, throat, skin, eg. measles) whereas bacterial infections tend to localize (one ear, lobe of lung, pointing abscess) — 'Lightwood's law'.

6. The primary duty of any hospital children's doctor is to discharge children therefrom.
7. Mother is right until proven otherwise.
8. One of the primary functions of tonsils is to get infected.
9. Inspection might better be considered as *observation*.
10. If you find one major malformation look for others: malformations tend to be multiple.
11. Students should not be systems specialists.

7. Maternal myths

While we are continually impressed by the correctness of maternal instincts there are certain myths that mothers persist in perpetrating. Below are some examples that students may meet — try compiling your own list from your clients.

1. Nose picking is associated with intestinal worms.
2. Laxatives will 'clear badness out of children'.
3. Strapping, strictures and mercurochrome will cure thumbsucking.
4. Worms are a cause of bedwetting (very rarely true).
5. A copper penny will cure umbilical hernias (they resolve themselves).
6. Goat's milk is good for eczema.
7. Breast fed babies are never obese (ask a student of medieval art — chubby cherubs abound).
8. Caries in primary teeth don't matter ('sweet tooths' carry on!).
9. Teething causes convulsions (teething produces teeth).
10. Early walking produces bow-legs.

8. Acrimonious acronyms

TORCH = toxoplasmosis, other, rubella, cytomegalovirus, herpes.
NTD   = neural tube defect.

CDH	=	congenital dislocated hips.
CHD	=	congenital heart disease.
FLK	=	'funny looking kid'; a term best avoided.
IRDS	=	idiopathic respiratory distress syndrome.
LBW	=	low birth weight.
VLBW	=	very low birth weight.
SGA	=	small for gestational age (sometimes called light for dates, small for dates).
IDM	=	infant of diabetic mother.
IVH	=	intraventricular haemorrhage.
CPAP	=	continuous positive airways pressure.
PEEP	=	positive end expiratory pressure.
IPPV	=	intermittent positive pressure ventilation.
NEC	=	necrotizing enterocolitis.
PFC	=	persistent fetal circulation.
BPD	=	broncho-pulmonary dysplasia.
RLF	=	retrolental fibroplasia.
TTN	=	transient tachypnoea of newborn.
TAPVD	=	total anomalous pulmonary venous drainage.
ZIG	=	zoster immune globulin.
DTP	=	diphtheria, tetanus, pertussis (also called 'triple antigen').
FAS	=	fetal alcohol syndrome.

We all use acronyms. Don't pepper your notes or your examination paper with too many of them. Remember that MI can stand for myocardial infarct, mitral incompetence, mental illness, or a well known motorway.

9. A–Z of eponyms

Alport's syndrome	=	congenital nephritis plus deafness.
Arnold–Chiari malformation	=	displacement of medulla and cerebellum into spinal canal.

Apert's syndrome	=	acrocephaly plus syndactyly.
Barlow's manoeuvre	=	technique of examining for congenitally dislocated hip.
Barr bodies	=	chromatin mass in cell nuclei.
Beckwith–Wiedemann syndrome	=	enlarged tongue, enlarged viscera, gigantism.
Berger's disease	=	IgA nephropathy.
Bright's disease (obsolete)	=	post-streptococcal glomerulonephritis.
Blackfan–Diamond syndrome	=	congenital pure red cell aplasia.
Caffey's disease	=	infantile cortical hyperostosis.
Cornelia de Lange's syndrome	=	mental and physical retardation, typical facies.
Criggler–Najjar syndrome	=	rare deficiency of glucuronyl transferase.
Dandy–Walker malformation	=	atresia of foramina of Magendie and Luschka.
Dennie–Morgan fold	=	double infraorbital fold in eczematous children.
DiGeorge syndrome	=	congenital aplasia of thethymus.
Duckett–Jones criteria	=	criteria for diagnosis of rheumatic fever.
Epstein's pearls	=	epithelial pearls on roof of mouth.
Erb's palsy	=	upper arm type of brachial palsy.
Fallot's tetrad	=	ventricular septal defect, pulmonary stenosis, right ventricular hypertrophy, overriding aorta.

Fanconi's syndrome	= phospho-gluco-aminoacid-bicarbonaturia, proximal tubular leak. Also known as de Toni–Debré–Fanconi syndrome.
Fanconi's anaemia	= congenital aplastic anaemia.
Gilbert's syndrome	= persistent unconjugated hyperbilirubinaemia.
Guillain–Barré syndrome	= ascending polyneuritis.
Henoch–Schönlein syndrome	= vasculitis, arthritis, nephritis, abdominal pain.
Hand-Schüller–Christian disease	= a form of histiocytosis with diabetes insipidus and bone lesions.
Hirschprung's disease	= colonic aganglionosis.
Kaposi's varicelliform eruption	= herpetic skin lesions in eczematous children.
Kawasaki's disease	= mucocutaneous lymph node syndrome.
Klinefelter's syndrome	= phenotype associated with XXY genotype.
Koplik's spots	= white spots on buccal mucosa in measles prodrome.
Laurence–Moon–Biedl syndrome	= polydactyly, obesity, mental retardation.
Louis–Bar syndrome	= ataxia telangiectasia.
Lowe's syndrome	= oculocerebrorenal syndrome.
Meckel's diverticulum	= aberrant ectopic gastric mucosa.
Marfan's syndrome	= dislocated lens, tall stature, weak aortic wall.
Noonan's syndrome	= XO phenotype in the male, pulmonary stenosis.

Ortolani test	=	for congenital hip dislocation.
Potter's facies	=	squashed newborn faces associated with oligohydramnios.
Reye's syndrome	=	acute encephalopathy and liver failure.
Ritter's disease	=	scalded skin syndrome.
Russell–Silver syndrome	=	triangular facies, short stature, body asymmetry.
Sprengel's deformity	=	congenital upward displacement of the scapula.
Treacher Collins sydrome	=	mandibulofacial dysostosis.
Von-Recklinghausen's disease (obsolescent)	=	neurofibromatotis.
Von Gierke's disease (obsolete)	=	glycogen storage disease.
Von Willebrand's disease (obsolescent)	=	Factor VIII deficiency.
Wilm's tumour	=	nephroblastoma.
Zellweger's sydrome	=	cerebrohepatorenal syndrome.

The above list is by no means exhaustive. Eponyms are abused entities and should be discarded when the true nature of the described entity or syndrome becomes clear. Happily we have ended our list with examples of obsolete or obsolescent eponyms. Much as we would all like to have a memorable eponymous syndrome, so-named children benefit when the syndrome is untangled and it's components elucidated. Do remember that what today's doctors label as, for example, Henoch-Schönlein syndrome, may not resemble what the good German doctors described a century ago.

There is a certain mystique about nobly named syndromes and doctors which failed to impress Matthew Arnold who wrote as follows:

> 'Nor bring to watch me cease to live,
> Some doctor full of phrase and fame,
> To shake his sapient head and give
> The ill man can not cure — a name'.

Eponymic syndromes might be described as a baptized collection of signs and symptoms awaiting confirmation.

Dublin has abandonded Grave's disease in favour of thyrotoxicosis, Guy's hospital has allowed glomerulonephritis to supplant Bright's disease and Corrigan's pulse has irrevocably collapsed.

10. Tips for the paediatric examination

Assessment in paediatrics now usually consists of in-course (continuous) assessment and end-of-course examination. It may include case studies, project presentation, written paper, multiple choice questionnaire, objective structured clinical examination, and oral.

The following remarks refer to the more traditional type of examination with a prepared long case, and one or more short, unprepared cases. The examiners want to know if you are competent and confident in handling children. They do not seek omniscience — if you don't know the answer to something, say so, rather than hazarding guesses.

Some simple commonsense rules to remember:

1. Extract from the mother or guardian all the information you can obtain. Remember that children with chronic conditions (heart disease, cystic fibrosis) can be remarkably informative. Don't give the child food or sweets without first checking with Sister or staff nurse.
2. Observe the child for the first few minutes before making physical contact. Note any observable clinical signs related to symptoms in the history. Assess the degree of illness (well, ill, quite ill). Comment on developmental status (alertness, social interaction, etc).

3. Above all, be gentle with the child despite your apprehension.

4. Don't forget to weigh and measure the child and plot on appropriate centile charts.

5. Perform a thorough systematic examination, leaving possibly unpleasant bits to the end.

6. Present the relevant positive historical factors first. Try to put the positive clinical findings in order of their importance. If you have come to a conclusion with which you are comfortable say so: 'This is Johnny Murphy, aged 5 years, who has features of Down's syndrome, has a murmur compatible with a ventricular septal defect, and has an abdominal scar consistent with repaired duodenal atresia'.

7. Suggest a differential diagnosis on the basis of positive clinical findings. If pressed for a possible diagnosis always 'back the favourite' and go for common conditions, avoiding rare conditions ('outside chances') unless very sure of them.

8. Don't make your examiners work unnecessarily — try to lead the discussion. If given the opportunity to reconsider your findings, be sure to avail of it. Examiners are usually trying to help, not to trip.

9. Relax, relax if possible. Your examiners are seeking confidence and competence. If you are well trained, you should have both attributes.

11. Alarm signals: ?non-accidental injury

Listed below is a selection of physical signs which may be suggestive of inflicted rather than accidental injuries:
- torn frenum in bottle fed infants
- black eyes in toddlers
- finger marks on cheeks
- petechiae on the pinna

- scratch marks
- teeth imprints anywhere
- punched out burns (?cigarettes)
- bruises in non-traumatic sites
- retinal haemorrhages
- perivaginal bruises
- Bruises of varying ages.

In addition the experienced observer may recognize as being alerting:

- 'frozen watchfulness' (a cold unemotional look)
- persistent gaze avoidance
- extremely unkempt appearance
- severe nappy rash.

12. Cliniquiz

1. Describe the features of finger clubbing. What are its causes in childhood?
2. What is sinus arrhythmia?
3. List 6 skills acquired by a 12-month-old infant.
4. Describe the rash of atopic eczema.
5. What are the features of an innocent/physiological/flow murmur?
6. Give 4 explanations for a large head in infancy.
7. What are (a) chorea, (b) cogwheel rigidity, (c) anasarca?
8. Clinically how might you distinguish laryngotracheo-bronchitis from epiglottitis?
9. What did (a) Kernig, (b) Koplik, (c) Korotkov describe?
10. What is the physiology of squatting in cyanotic heart disease?
11. Why do babies with respiratory difficulty grunt?
12. What are (a) pulsus paradoxus, (b) pulsus alternans, (c) collapsing pulse?
13. Why do infants become mottled when ill?

14. What is the purpose of shivering?
15. Think of 5 explanations for an acute limp in 3-year-old child.
16. List 5 causes of meningism other than meningitis.
17. Which is the diastolic pressure point — phase 4 (muffling) or phase 5 (disappearance of sounds)?
18. Give 4 causes of acute wheezing in infants.
19. List 10 patterns of injury suggestive of non-accidental injury.
20. Name some drugs which may be associated with hirsutism.

Recommended reading

Paediatric texts

Apley J 1979 Paediatrics, 2nd edn. Ballière-Tindall, London. Read the first few chapters for paediatric philosophy.

Habel A 1982 Aids to paediatrics. Churchill Livingstone, Edinburgh. Helpful hints and lists unlimited. Postgraduate emphasis.

Habel A 1986 Aids to paediatrics for undergraduates. Churchill Livingstone, Edinburgh.

Hull D, Johnson D I 1987 Essential paediatrics, 2nd edn. Churchill Livingstone, Edinburgh. The most current basic test.

Illingworth R S 1986 The normal child, 9th edn. Churchill Livingstone, Edinburgh. A well of information.

King M, King F, Martodipoero S 1978 Primary child care. Oxford University Press. Essential reading for electives in developing countries.

Sheridan M D 1975 From birth to five years, 3rd edn. NEFR — Nelson, Winsdor. Child development made simple and interesting.

Picture books

Bain J, Cater P, Morton R 1985 Colour atlas of mouth, throat and ear disorders in children. MTP Press, Lancaster.

Milner R G D, Heber S M 1986 Diagnostic picture tests in paediatrics. Wolfe, London.

O'Doherty N 1982 The battered child: recognition in primary care. Baillière-Tindall, London. A pictorial introduction to child abuse.

O'Doherty N 1985 Atlas of the Newborn , 2nd edn. MTP Press, Lancaster. A good compilation of neonatal variations.

Spitz L, Steiner G M, Zachary R B 1981 A colour atlas of paediatric surgical diagnosis. Wolfe, London.

Thomas R, Harvey D 1984 Colour Aids: Neonatology. Churchill Livingstone, Edinburgh

Thomas R, Harvey D 1986 Colour Aids: Paediatrics. Churchill Livingstone, Edinburgh. Easy reading and good pictures.

Verbov J 1982 Colour atlas of paediatric dermatology. MTP Press, Lancaster. Pictures of skins are worth thousands of words.

Reference texts

Buckler J M H 1979 A reference manual of growth and development. Blackwell, Oxford. Measures up well to growth information.

Goodman R M, Gorlin R J 1983 The malformed infant and child. Oxford University Press, Oxford. Excellent line drawings, concise text.

Smith D W 1981 Recognizable patterns of human deformation. Saunders, Philadelphia.

Smith D W 1982 Recognizable patterns of human malformation, 3rd edn. Saunders, Philadelphia. A superb reference on dysmorphology.

Tanner J M, Whitehouse R H 1982 Atlas of children's growth. Academic Press, London. A library luxury. Stunningly detailed.

Clinical signs

Koop C E 1976 Visible and palpable lesions in children. Grune and Stratton, New York. A useful selection from a skilled surgeon.

Macleod J Munro J 1986 Clinical examination, 7th edn. Churchill Livingstone, Edinburgh.

Pappworth M H 1984 A primer of medicine, 5th edn. Butterworths, London. Not only for neurology, but much more . . . . .

Index